Fifty Years a Doctor

The Journey of Sickness and Health, Four Plagues
and the Pandemic

Ronald Halweil, MD

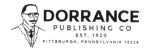
DORRANCE
PUBLISHING CO
EST. 1920
PITTSBURGH, PENNSYLVANIA 15238

Dorrance Publishing Co
585 Alpha Drive
Pittsburgh, PA 15238
Visit our website at *www.dorrancebookstore.com*

ISBN: 978-1-6853-7183-8
eISBN: 978-1-6853-7725-0

Fifty Years a Doctor

The Journey of Sickness and Health, Four Plagues
and the Pandemic

I would not have been able to write this book without the love, support, wisdom and inspiration of my beautiful wife, children and grandchildren.

This book could not have been completed without the artistic and technical support of Gil Ferrer and Carlos Ferrer. I would also like to thank Carrington Morris for her advice and editing.

Ronald Halweil MD
ronhalweilmd@gmail.com

Table of Contents

Introduction

Why would anyone take the time to write a book unless there was a compulsion to tell people an interesting story. This story is about a medical doctor's fifty-plus-year journey through medicine, health and health care in a very different time than today. The things I saw as a medical and surgical practitioner in an era without the technological advances we have today. The four plagues I saw before the recent pandemic. Things happen much faster nowadays, and what used to be normal can now seem unusual, and yet it was valid, and worked at that time, just as things we take for granted about health and health care today may be looked upon as primitive in the future.

My journey in the medical field started as a newborn and is still ongoing as a senior doctor. This is a snapshot of my era. The history of medicine predates civilization and is still being recorded as new developments and discoveries are made daily, and yet humans, *Homo sapiens*, are the same as they ever were, as are so many of their health problems.

Sometimes it feels like every new advance is paired with a loss of older wisdom, as if there is no room for the old with the new, and I think this is a big mistake that causes needless suffering and premature death. My hope is that you will enjoy this story and learn something of value from it.

Chapter One - Fifty Years a Doctor: The Beginning

I was destined to be a doctor.

Shortly after my birth, my mom's dad saw me and said, "He will be a doctor," and my mom did everything she could to honor his wish for me. A noble profession, and there was a shortage of doctors in the America of my youth.

A great career and a good income. I would be my own boss, working for myself and my patients. It was a perfect profession for a bright student with interests in the sciences, biology, chemistry, physics.

I had interviews at several prestigious medical schools, but the ones that accepted me could not give me a full scholarship. I accepted the excellent New York State Medical School in Brooklyn, which based tuition on family income, giving me a very low tuition. To this day I do not regret going to SUNY Downstate, where I got a superb medical education over four years.

My specialty

I considered general practice like my family doctor, whom I admired ever since early childhood, but this was the age of specialization, and after spending time in all the medical and surgical specialties, I was torn between obstetrics and gynecology (ob-gyn) and the burgeoning field of microsurgery being used by ear, nose and throat doctors to restore hearing.

I always enjoyed microscopy, and I was fascinated by this new form of surgery. Also, ENT, as it was known, was a field that treated all ages and sexes, and took care of medical and surgical problems, so I could be a family doctor for this area of the body.

Unfortunately for me, the obstetrics custom at that time was to see a patient when she first became pregnant and then be her doctor until she delivered a baby with your help and guidance, even in the middle of the night. This was troubling to me since I really needed to get a good night's sleep to be my best, and one of our favorite obstetrical teachers told us that once in his career he was in the hospital with a different patient in labor for forty consecutive days and nights.

Careful investigation taught me that ENT doctors had a good chance of getting a full night's sleep most of the time. In addition to microsurgery, there was plastic surgery of the face, which appealed to my artistic interests, and that was how otolaryngology won and delivering babies lost.

To qualify for a residency in ENT in the '60s, you first had to complete a one-year internship and one year of general surgery. I interned in internal medicine, with an elective in psychiatry, at Metropolitan Hospital and Flower 5th Avenue Hospital. I was fortunate enough to have selected my general surgery training in a unique program called the Honolulu Integrated Surgical Residency, which rotated through the three main hospitals in Honolulu.

The biggest hospital, where we spent the most time, was the Queen's Hospital, donated to the people of Honolulu in1859 by Queen Emma and King Kamehameha IV of Hawaii to help the native people of Hawaii who were suffering and dying from a recent epidemic of smallpox plus all the other infections inadvertently brought to Hawaii by Europeans and other non-Polynesian visitors.

St. Francis Hospital was the Chinese hospital, and Kuakini was the Japanese hospital and the smallest of the three, but with the best food and the best "on call" room.

In 1967 the Queen's Hospital became Queen's Medical Center, but everyone still called it Queen's Hospital.

My three-year otolaryngology residency at the New York Eye and Ear Infirmary had already been confirmed before I left for Hawaii. In addition to the obvious benefits of spending a year in Hawaii, the hospitals there paid twice as much as the NYC hospitals! But I never expected to have one of the greatest educational experiences of my life there, as I worked with experienced surgeons in a program with a shortage of residents. This meant I was very involved in every operation, rather than being a second or third assistant at the operating table at a large New York City hospital.

This was an era of medicine when the fabulous imaging technologies of today were nonexistent. There was no CAT scan or MRI to reveal the hidden spaces of the human body, not even ultrasound to help determine if a swelling was benign or malignant.

This was a time when the surgeon was called upon to make the diagnosis from patient history, physical examination, and personal experience, and often that needed a closer inspection, meaning an exploratory operation, and possibly a life-saving procedure being performed at the same time.

I worked in general surgery, which was the most valuable surgical field because a general surgeon could handle the widest range of problems that called for surgical treatment. This was the time before general surgery had completed its splitting into many different subspecialties. If there was a crisis, wartime, accidents, a fire, an earthquake, mass shooting, or any other catastrophe, you would hope a general surgeon was readily available to save lives.

The younger general surgeons were very popular with the nurses and other young women working at the Queen's Hospital. They were the rock stars of the hospital, and I quickly learned that they all had "hospital girlfriends" and at the same time had wives at home and maybe children as well. Yes, they were the rock stars.

Within a short period of time, I found myself in the same position with a beautiful radiology instructor. We met for a light breakfast every morning before surgery at the Queen's Hospital outdoor café and developed a loving relationship.

I also worked in gynecology, urology, neurosurgery, trauma surgery, ear, nose and throat surgery, vascular surgery, thoracic surgery, head and neck surgery, thyroid surgery, and plastic and cosmetic surgery. I learned how to harvest different thicknesses of skin to be used for grafting injured people, especially at the Queen's Hospital burn center.

One episode on the first day of my surgical training at Queen's stands out as the most unexpected event. The case was gallbladder surgery. The three of us at the operating table were dressed in our sterile gowns with sterile gloves and facial masks, the senior surgeon, the scrub nurse, and me. No one could see what anyone looked like with these surgical costumes.

The surgeon welcomed me to the hospital and got my name and where I was trained. Then he handed me the scalpel. I was shocked since I had no formal surgical training. He must have assumed that my recently completed internship was a surgical internship, which was most common with first-year surgical residents. I turned the scalpel around and handed it back to the surgeon. This was unprecedented, and though I could not see the expression on his face, I can imagine the look of astonishment. This may be the first time ever a surgical resident handed the scalpel back to the surgeon.

I explained to him that I had been a medical intern and that I had a residency in ENT waiting for me when this year of surgical residency was completed. As the operation proceeded, I was the first assistant and would hold a retractor to expose the operative site and a suction or sponge to remove blood from the operative site.

The operation was proceeding smoothly. The anesthesiologist was keeping the patient still and the scrub nurse was handing different instruments to the surgeon as he called for them. When the scrub nurse brushed my thigh with her body. I took that for an accidental move and thought nothing of it. Then it happened again, and her thigh rubbed against mine. I was twenty-six years old and surmised that this was an intentional move on her part and I reciprocated. I quickly looked at her and saw a wisp of blonde hair protruding from her surgical cap, and that she had blue eyes. I recorded this information carefully. The operation went smoothly and I helped with the suturing at the end using scissors to cut the ends of sutures as they were tied.

After surgery, doctors and nurses retired to a spacious communal lounge to relax, have coffee and gossip. When I got to the lounge I was looking for a blonde with blue eyes, and then I saw three scrub nurses with blonde hair and blue eyes sitting together and talking and laughing!

Months later I found out which nurse had been in the OR that first day. She was very friendly when we met, but I was unable to accept her very tempting offer to spend a weekend with her and her two lovely roommates at their house since I already had a steady girl-friend at the hospital, and a wife at home!

The superior training I got in this exceptional training program gave me great confidence entering my first of three years of specialized training in otolaryngology. I doubt if any of my friends who stayed in NYC had the varied and extensive surgical training that I had.

Chapter Two - Memories of Medical School

For the first time in my life I was not living in the Brooklyn apartment with my parents and younger sister where we all lived since my grade school years. I stayed home when I went to Brooklyn College, a short commute from my family home. College was not all consuming. Some days there were only a few hours of classes and the rest of the time was mine. Obviously there was homework, but even after that a large part of the day was still mine and I had opportunities to work at various jobs and earn spending money.

Rent and groceries were not an issue while I lived with my parents. I even got a check twice a year from a New York State academic scholarship. Medical school was a whole other experience. There was rent, sharing a basement apartment in the East Flatbush area of Brooklyn with another medical student, and I had to feed myself and clean up after myself after long days in classes and cadaver dissection lab. This was a real problem for someone with very little money.

I had some savings from my college scholarship and from a summer job at a camp in New Hampshire the previous year, and I did get a small allowance from my parents. I had to be very careful about how I spent my money for food. This was the poorest time of my life and the loneliest. If I was to learn all that I was taught in classes and in our textbooks there was little time for socializing, and dating would be a burden for me on my very limited budget.

One memory that stands out from this basement apartment is...
THE RATS!

I may not have cleaned the kitchen well enough when I cooked my own dinners, and one night I heard noises in the kitchen, dishes and pans moving. I had seen rats in the area around the house, probably related to new construction and disturbances of the homes of different animals, rats included. I didn't fear the rats since I thought they would be too timid to invade my sleeping space. Boy was I wrong.

One night while in a deep sleep I felt something crawling on my back and instantly I was wide awake and knew that a rat was on my back. I sat up so fast that the rat went flying off me and onto the linoleum floor where I heard frantic scratching as the rat regained its balance and ran away to safety. That was the end of my sleep for the night. Within two days, I moved to an above-ground apartment nearby and my fellow med students helped me move the few things I needed to take while the landlady cursed me and shouted that she didn't have rats. Shortly after that, I met a woman who would become my wife and we were able to move to even better accommodations.

One cold winter morning we had to leave the warmth of the medical school to get to Kings County Hospital across the street for "rounding" with attendings. We didn't have our full winter clothing on since it was only across the street, but we moved quickly to get into the warm entrance of the hospital. As we got near the hospital I noticed a large group of people, mostly of color, huddled near another hospital entrance which was not open. They appeared older and most were bent over in their heavy winter clothing. Later in the day I asked a security guard about them and he said that they were waiting for the clinics to open and usually arrive early to be seen first. It seemed cruel to me that these shivering older people could not wait inside the warm hospital on this very cold winter morning.

People of my generation say that they have clear memories of where they were and what they were doing on the day President Kennedy was assassinated. I was in the dissection room, where our class was divided into groups of three or four students sharing a cadaver to learn anatomy. That day we had our cadavers propped up to learn about the perineum and the anus and its muscles when we heard some people in the hallway shouting that our young President Kennedy had been shot. Within a few minutes we all knew this terrible thing and could no longer do the mundane dissection of the cadaver's bottom.

We covered up our cadavers and joined the crowds in the hallways to commiserate and get details and find out if our president would live.

Football with a heart

Almost all the medical students in our class were in their early twenties. Sometimes the work we did and the hours we kept were too much and we had to let off some steam. This happened one evening following a particularly long and difficult day in dissection lab where the smell of formaldehyde never went away, a strong chemical smell that we now know is considered very unhealthy and probably carcinogenic. We "lost it" as a group when one of the students tossed a cadaver heart to another student and a "football" game started with cheering and running between the cadaver tables.

Our excitement was contagious and loud. After a few minutes we got caught when a senior physician in our training program hearing all the shouting entered the lab and reprimanded us for being disrespectful to the cadaver and acting in a childish way. We all regained our professional demeanor and apologized. After that we covered up the cadavers, left the lab and went our separate ways to our homes.

The long hours in class every day and the studying we had to do at night while we were tired was a problem with me and other students. I had actually never had an "all-nighter" in college, where a group studied together and lost a night's sleep, but I knew I was falling behind in my studying in order to get enough sleep. When I mentioned this to other students, a few said that I should try a small dose of Dexedrine, a commonly used stimulant and appetite suppressant to help me study, when I was tired and that it had helped them. I was curious about this and asked how I could get this medication.

I was told that a drugstore near the hospital had a druggist who would sell Dexedrine pills to medical students without a prescription and at a discount.

The next day I went to see the druggist, and sure enough after I told him that I was a medical student he sold me ten 5mg pills for $1.50. The next evening, after another long day in classes, I found myself too tired to study, so I took one of the pills and was able to have two very productive hours of studying that felt like I was as alert as I would normally be in the morning. Other students who I spoke with also said that sometimes after taking the Dexedrine pill it would be hard to fall asleep, and I would probably need a mild sleeping pill that I could get from the same druggist. So I went back to the friendly druggist and he sold me ten low-dose phenobarbital pills, a common sleeping pill, for $1.

I was not used to taking medicines, but I tried that, too, and found that I slept well but woke up groggy in the morning, something I was not used to feeling. I mentioned this to the older medical student in the basement apartment we shared and he recommended not taking these medications and that he had a car accident one morning because the sleeping pill effect lasted much longer than he expected. So I took his advice and stopped taking these pills and went back to my regular study schedule.

Delivering babies at night

Part of our training in obstetrics and gynecology involved overnight work in "labor and delivery." Our training program in this specialty was robust, since ob-gyn was one of the major hallmarks of this medical school. We were all seasoned in our obstetrical work after being attentive to our mentors, and now was the time when we became the "doctors" and were given patients in labor to take care of until delivery and the immediate postpartum period.

We were not alone in this department since there were experienced obstetrical nurses available to help us and senior ob-gyn residents on call if we needed even more help. Acting as the doctor in charge of this important service boosted our confidence as "almost doctors." We had already done a full day's work in class by this late hour and were looking forward to our bedroom which consisted of seven beds lined up in a small room facing the hospital laundry with the giant thundering steam chimney that never got quiet.

After we had finished our last delivery and found no immediate postpartum problems and completed our handwritten chart notes, we could go to bed to get some sleep before the obstetrical rounds with the professors in the early morning, just a few hours away.

As each med student finished his work, he would go to the bedroom, pick a vacant bed and nod off. But there was a problem one night. That night there were more students than beds. It was always assumed that there would probably be one or two med students still caring for women in labor and no need for an eighth bed in that crowded space, but after all seven beds were occupied there was one last student finishing up after delivery, and when he got to the bedroom he couldn't find a bed! No one could give up a narrow bed or share a bed, so this unfortunate student had to go back to labor and delivery and find a chair to sleep on, but not before loud cursing and kicking the bedroom wall.

My worst illness

Our favorite internist and chairman of the internal medicine department was lecturing us on sensitivity to patients' suffering when they have a serious illness. He stressed that our sensitivity would increase as we got older and had more life experiences, and then he added a wish that every one of us should have a serious illness from which we would have a complete recovery. I thought that was a strange thing to wish on us and quickly forgot it.

We were scheduled to begin our pediatric rotation with a visit to the pediatric infectious disease ward at Kings County Hospital, and the pediatrician attending told us to call our moms and check to see if we had all the childhood diseases, like chickenpox, mumps, measles, and German measles. I called my mom that evening and she laughed and was emphatic that I had everything. I myself remembered my childhood suffering with them, too, especially the chickenpox I had when I was six which caused me to miss the first three weeks of first grade.

The pediatric infectious ward at Kings County was full of crying children and bad smells as our "attending" took us around to see the various different diseases. She stopped at one crib and picked up a crying child and asked if we knew what this child had. I said measles when I saw the rash, and she handed me the baby and asked me to pass her around so we all had the experience of holding a feverish and crying infant. Then we saw other cases of infectious diseases and we were all relieved to finally exit this awful smelling ward of crying children. Remember, this was an era before routine vaccinations for these "childhood" diseases were available.

The lectures on pediatric illnesses were conducted in the usual conference rooms, and we did our note taking and studying as usual because we would be tested at the end of the pediatric rotation. About a week later I woke up with a headache, something I rarely get, and I felt chilled as well, but I quickly got dressed as I usually do and went to the lecture hall with my friends to start our daily education. My headaches and chills continued and I told my friends, who said it was probably a cold, although I was not sneezing or coughing. I took aspirin to relieve my symptoms, but it didn't help much except to bring my temperature down a little. When I continued to feel sick with a headache and chills the next day, I decided to go to the student health doctor for an exam and possible treatment. He didn't find anything wrong with me except for a fever and said we will have to wait to see if this gets worse. He recommended that I return to see him in a day or two if my symptoms persisted. As a medical student I was already thinking of the worst things this illness could be, and my friends were also thinking of a differential diagnosis, like leukemia or Hodgkin's disease. My close friends were caring, but things don't stand still in medical school, and we continued to attend our classes as usual.

Finally, I noticed some spots on my throat while I was brushing my teeth and that made me think I had caught something from the children's infectious ward. I returned to the student health physician, who told me I had measles, and I was relieved that I could forget about leukemia as a diagnosis. He then asked me if I wanted to be admitted to the children's ward at Kings County. I thought he was joking and said, "of course not." He told me that I would become very ill and would need lots of help through the illness, and I said my wife and mom would be able to help me at home. My wife was working to support us and would be away during the day, but my mom would be able to take care of me and also my grandmother and my closest aunt and they worked out a schedule. I soon found out why all the babies were crying.

Within a day of the diagnosis my fever increased and I developed alternating diarrhea and vomiting. My mom put a large bowl on the bed for me to vomit into because I had become too weak to keep running to the toilet, and she would clean the bowl every time I threw up and help me to the toilet when I had diarrhea. I also had a bad sore throat, a running nose, a cough and an earache, and my headache never let up. I understood that the measles virus was multiplying and affecting every part of my body and that my immune system was producing antibodies as quickly as possible but not fast enough to end my misery.

I had no appetite but I was always thirsty, and though swallowing was painful, I drank as much ginger ale without bubbles as I could so that I wouldn't get dehydrated and need to go to the pediatric ward at Kings County for intravenous hydration. I was very grateful for the work of the four women who cared for me day and night. Over the next two weeks I started to improve and my diarrhea and vomiting left, then my fever broke and my headaches ceased. I had more strength and could walk around the apartment, my grandmother and aunt no longer needed to take care of me, and I was able to eat the food left by my wife and mom. But there was one more discomfort that the measles had for me, and that was severe itching all over my body, and that lasted for several days.

Finally I was well enough to go outside and consider a trip to medical school to restart my studies. My home scale showed that I had lost twenty pounds in these two and a half weeks, something I suspected when my pants fell down unless I would really tighten my belt. I went to the pediatrics department office to talk about my long absence, and the same doctor who handed me the measles baby was there to greet me and ask how I was feeling. I gave her a little synopsis of weeks of misery, and pointed to my loose pants, but said that I was feeling much better now. Then she told me that I had missed too much of the pediatric rotation and would need to do it over again.

At that point I told her that after what I went through I could not conceive of doing this and I might die from another infection, and in any case I should get honors for my in-depth personal instruction in childhood diseases. She reluctantly accepted this. I would not have to repeat the course, but she did not give me honors for the experience I had. I was still curious as to why I had no immunity to measles if I had every disease like my mom said.

I contacted my old family doctor who was my mom's obstetrician, our family's general practitioner and my pediatrician, and he did have records from that period of my life. Apparently when I was exposed to measles as a young child, there was a new medical innovation to prevent the measles that had gained some popularity in pediatric practice. This involved an injection of gamma globulin, a mixed blood immune cell product that would grant limited immunity to many infectious diseases. In that era, and even today, measles could cause severe permanent health problems and even death, so that any way to avoid this disease was considered worthwhile. And that explained why I had no immunity twenty years later to that little measles baby. My medical school friends were happy to see me and were amazed at my weight loss. So apparently I was the only student to take the advice of the chief of internal medicine and have a serious and painful disease and get a full recovery.

To this day, that was the worst illness I have ever had.

Chapter Three - The Smoking Epidemic

Smoking

My mom was a smoker, a heavy smoker. Two packs a day, every day, unless she was sick. My dad didn't smoke and he was the exception since most adults in America at that time smoked. When I was growing up in the '50s I wanted to smoke when I got older. I helped my mom by running to the local candy store with the 60 cents she gave me to buy her two packs of Chesterfields regular and get a comic book for myself with the extra dime. I was so proud to help my mother. Mom smoked everywhere in our small apartment, and in the morning I would see an ashtray of cigarette butts at her bedside, too. She smoked in the car with me and my baby sister, and I was amazed that she could light a cigarette while she was driving.

By the time I was ten I wanted to smoke to appear older and more sophisticated.

By age twelve I was full grown and looked like I was in my late teens so I was able to buy a pack of cigarettes by myself and try smoking. It made me dizzy and nauseated, but I knew that if I continued smoking I would get over these side effects. But it wasn't working out. I would get ashes on my pants and little burn holes and I never got over the nausea or lightheadedness, so I stopped smoking.

I was an underweight baby at birth, the result of my mom's smoking during pregnancy. Years later, in medical school, our obstetrics textbook had a passage about pregnancy and smoking. It said that it might be too traumatic for a pregnant woman to stop smoking completely so we should encourage less smoking, rather than no smoking. This was followed by the information that smokers have smaller babies at birth and this makes delivery easier, which is a good thing. I remember a special edition of *Life* magazine that included fifty years of photos of the featured people on each week's cover: All of them were smoking, something, a cigarette, a pipe or a cigar, another example of the pervasiveness of this addictive activity.

Cigarettes and other tobacco products plus the advertising agencies that cleverly promoted them were important parts of the American economy, and the federal, state and local taxes on these products were very important and helped with government financing. There was a delicate balance between low cigarette taxes not bringing in enough revenue and high taxes discouraging smokers and creating a black market in cigarettes which yielded no taxation revenue. I remember the clever TV ads of white-coated actors representing doctors explaining why one brand of cigarette was better than other brands because of the way it was manufactured. Even the prestigious and powerful AMA (American Medical Association) benefited from cigarettes by running similar ads.

Everyone knew there were deleterious health effects from smoking, but the occasional sore throat or the "smoker's cough" or hoarse voice were considered an incidental inconvenience and not significant enough to give up a very pleasurable habit. The nicotine in tobacco is a well-known stimulant and is addictive. Growing up I heard cigarettes referred to as "coffin nails" well before any professional, scientific or governmental pronouncements.

The well-known and respected Canadian internist, Dr. William Osler, at the beginning of the 20th century had a grand rounds to show medical students and other hospital personnel a case they may never see again: a case of lung cancer! As the years passed, there was research and other evidence that prolonged use of smoked tobacco products were very detrimental and could shorten life span. I remember seeing some of these experiments shown on TV news, where tobacco smoking tars placed on the backs of mice would grow cancerous tumors.

In 1957 the U.S. Surgeon General made the first official governmental statement that "smoking" could cause cancer. Some people stopped smoking after this announcement, but not too many. Habits and addictions are hard to break.

Our first lectures in medical school in 1963 were about smoking and alcohol.

At that time nearly one-quarter of the class were smokers, and our lecture hall often smelled of lighted cigarettes since there were few prohibitions against smoking anywhere you wanted—there were even smoking rooms in hospitals for the convenience of the patients. Our professors presented slide after slide of x-rays showing lung cancer and pathology slides of what lung cancer looked like under the microscope. And they lectured on all the new evidence of smoking causing cancer. We had these lectures for several consecutive days, and at the end of this intense period of lectures on the dangers of smoking there were fewer smokers in the auditorium! These lectures on the dangers of smoking were followed by another series of lectures and presentations on the dangers of drinking alcohol to excess.

The focus of these lectures was on alcoholism and the danger to the brain and liver. I was impressed that our first teaching in med school would be so topical and personal instead of focusing on a rare condition, and that there had already been a positive change in the lives of our student body after these lectures. It's sad to think of all the deaths and miseries that could have been prevented if the doctors and the AMA, and the FDA and all the other governmental agencies had been more proactive in alerting the populace to the problems of smoking.

My mom died of cancer. When she got the diagnosis of metastatic cancer, she finally stopped smoking and regretted that her lifelong habit prevented her from having more time with her young grandchildren. Sadly, the smoking epidemic is still with us.

A new industry has developed around smoking cessation. Nicotine patches and nicotine chewing gum are available without a prescription, but my patients would complain that they were too expensive and they couldn't afford them. Then there is the prescription drug Chantix, which needs a doctor's visit to get a prescription and which could have serious side effects such as headaches, dizziness, constipation, suicidal thoughts, hallucinations, and anxiety disorder. There is even help for cigarette smokers over the telephone which is free.

And yet the epidemic continues.

When I was a teaching "attending" at the New York Eye and Ear Infirmary in the new millennium, I met a medical student from Australia who was taking an ENT elective. I asked him about how his country handled the smoking epidemic, and he told me that cigarettes in Australia were very expensive. I told him that they were very expensive here, too, at $10 a pack in New York City, and he said they were $20 (U.S. dollars) a pack in Australia and that really cut down the amount of smoking. I said that would work here, too.

Obviously there are many ways to reduce smoking but apparently we don't have the will to make it happen, and that means more cancer, more COPD (chronic obstructive pulmonary disease), and more misery and premature deaths for the addicted smokers, as well as more secondhand smoke for the friends and children of smokers.

Chapter Four - Internship

After graduating from medical school we all take internships, which are a one-year program of being a real doctor treating real people with real health problems. Unfortunately working as doctors just out of medical school with lots of book knowledge but not much actual experience treating patients and without an attending doctor nearby is not the best way to learn acute or even chronic medical care.

For me and most of the young doctors that I knew from medical school, this was scary and stressful especially when we covered the emergency room at night. We were told that there were doctors who could be called if we needed them, but if we were confronted with acute problems that had to be treated right away, this didn't leave time for a phone call. One other big stress of this nighttime doctoring experience was our tired, sleep-deprived state, where our functioning was different than it would be in the daytime. My internship was in internal medicine in a large city hospital on the Upper East Side of Manhattan, Metropolitan Hospital, and a short time at Flower 5th Avenue Hospital, which was like a private hospital opposite Central Park, also on the Upper East Side of Manhattan.

On my first day being the only doctor in the emergency room at Metropolitan Hospital, I was confronted by a loud group of seven men carrying another man into the emergency room while they were all shouting at me in Spanish. They laid a young man with a blue-tinged face on the exam table while they continued shouting at me. I could see that he wasn't breathing well and started searching for an endotracheal tube when the ER nurse handed me a full syringe and told me it was a heroin overdose and I had to find a vein and quickly inject this Nalline (a chemical cousin to Narcan) or he's going to die. I had no trouble finding a good vein and gave him the full dose.

Within one minute the semi-comatose man started breathing and moving on the exam table, at which point the group of men started laughing and lifted their friend and rushed him out of the hospital before I had any time to fill out a chart or even get his name. And that was my first day as a solo doctor in the emergency room.

I remember seeing a middle-aged man with chest discomfort but no shortness of breath. He told me that this started after eating a large Italian dinner with three glasses of wine. He laughed when he said this has happened before but sometimes he just can't resist all the spicy food and wine. I treated him for heartburn/indigestion after finding normal pulse, blood pressure and chest sounds and sent him home. That man returned the next morning and was diagnosed with a heart attack and was admitted into the hospital, and I was told that I had missed the diagnosis even though I had no experience with all the various presentations of acute heart attacks.

On another night, a tall man with bright yellow pants and orange jacket and a large fancy hat entered the ER with a sad young woman attractively dressed with deep chest cleavage and a miniskirt and high heels. The nurse who admitted her said she had vaginal pain on intercourse, something we call "dyspareunia." When I put the whole picture together, I realized that the flashy-dressed man was a pimp and his best prostitute was out of action on a Saturday night due to vaginal pain. I reached the ob-gyn resident on call and told him the story. He understood and said he would be right down.

Several times I saw teenage girls with high fever and foul-smelling vaginal discharge and the nurse told me it was septic abortion and I found out this awful thing was common in this era without access to legal abortion, and young women had to try anything to get rid of the unwanted child. These septic abortions were immediately hospitalized on the ob-gyn floor.

We also had to take care of patients on the regular hospital floors who had been kept in hospital beds for many days, weeks or even months. For these patients we tried to determine the cause of their medical problems, so that they could get the right treatment, recover and be discharged from the hospital. We did blood tests daily and x-rays and presented their cases to the internist attending physicians. These attendings would then go over the medical records, get a short history from the patients, perform a physical exam and finally give a diagnosis and recommend a treatment program. We followed everything they recommended, and if the patient expired, we went to the morgue to watch the autopsy and noted that the expert's diagnosis was wrong nearly 50 percent of the time. This was an era where we had no CAT scans or MRIs to look inside the sick bodies and provide us with information to get a better medical diagnosis.

And then there was the eleven-year-old boy who approached me in the ER before he was registered and asked if he should take the new opioid drug methadone to get him off heroin. He told me his "drug pusher" could get it for him. I told him to stop all the drugs and got him a pediatric appointment for the next day. How sad was this? No eleven-year-old should ever have a problem like this.

One night on call I was asked to pronounce a male patient "dead." I had never been asked to do this before and was a little apprehensive since there were so many stories about patients waking up minutes or hours after being "pronounced," but the nurse with this old man said there was no doubt in her mind that he had died. I went up to the motionless body and looked for signs of breathing and then felt for a carotid artery pulse, and there was none. Then I listened to the chest for heart or breath sounds and they were absent. I also checked his eyes with a pocket flashlight and there was no response. I pronounced him dead and signed the papers, and yet still felt uneasy as I walked away. Most of the time in the ER involved less complicated cases like sore throats, earaches, colds and coughs and a surprisingly large number of hepatitis cases, as well as facial trauma from sports or fights.

After a while I started feeling more comfortable in my role as ER doctor. But then one day I developed a fever with stomach cramps and diarrhea and weakness and was sent home by an ER attending to recover. I was sure that I had hepatitis. Though I never had dark urine or jaundice and my fever and bowel problems were gone quickly, still

I felt weak. I went to the hospital staff health department and told the doctor about the fever and my fatigue problems. On examination the only findings were enlarged neck lymph nodes, which could be a sign of mononucleosis, a common viral infection in my age group that could cause weakness and fatigue.

I was told to rest at home for another week before returning to work. The fatigue never left and I was admitted to Flower Fifth Avenue Hospital for a more intensive workup. But even after three days in a hospital bed with blood tests and x-rays, there were no signs of serious illness and I was advised to return to work or risk having to repeat the internship. I discussed this with my wife and we decided I should go back to work and rest whenever I could.

The next few months were very difficult for me but I tried hard even though I always felt like I could go to sleep easily at any moment if I could lie down. The diagnosis of chronic fatigue syndrome was mentioned, but most doctors did not believe it was a real disease. Some of the other interns accepted my problems and helped me when they could by taking over one of my "on calls," while others thought I was malingering and were often disrespectful to me.

Finally when the winter was over I started feeling less fatigue, and by May I felt normal again. I completed my internship and was excited about my upcoming surgical residency in Hawaii. Today chronic fatigue syndrome is an accepted diagnosis that tends to follow a febrile infection. All in all I would have to say that the internship year was the most difficult and stressful part of my entire medical career, with long hours, sleep deprivation and inadequate attending supervision, plus my "mystery illness." A highlight of the internship was the elective in psychiatry, a less strenuous time in medicine where I was usually surrounded by several residents and not alone when there were complications. I also had a good friend during this time and we often spent lunchtime together and even socialized with our wives as couples and enjoyed his musical skills as he played his guitar and sang Bob Dylan songs.

I certainly hope that there have been improvements in the conduct of the internship so that better care for the patient and less stress for the young doctor have become the standards, and I'm sure that the improved diagnostics of the high-tech scans have been a big help.

Chapter Five - A Unique Residency

It took me years to fully realize what a unique residency program I had enjoyed in my one-year general surgical training in Honolulu. Early in this residency we had state-mandated education in leprosy. All the new doctors had to visit the Hawaiian leper colony on the island of Molokai for the tutorial and to see people with the disease.

We learned that leprosy, also called Hansen's disease, had been curable with antibiotics since 1940, and that all the people living on Molokai were cured but had many facial and body deformities and preferred to live with people like themselves, and they were supported by the State of Hawaii.

After spending most of a day on Molokai, we were relieved to learn that leprosy was not very contagious. Contrary to common thinking that a great residency program had to be at a large teaching hospital, the integrated surgical program was better because there were fewer residents, so you were not lost in a crowd of medical students, interns and residents.

In this residency program in small hospitals with many good surgeons, who were very attentive with one-on-one instruction to the young interns and residents, I had the opportunity to see the many different ways that skilled surgeons operated. As an example, in general surgery at some point a large incision had to be made into a patient's body. The most common area that we operated on was the abdominal area, and I saw several techniques for dealing with the bleeding that would naturally take place when a knife penetrates skin and flesh.

One day I assisted on an abdominal surgery performed with the common method of clamping each small blood vessel that was oozing blood from the incision and then cauterizing those vessels. Once all of the bleeding had stopped the surgery would progress. This technique seemed obvious and certainly controlled the bleeding problem. But then on the following day, with a different surgeon, I saw a totally different approach to the problem of incisional bleeding. In this case the surgeon used lap pads (pads to control bleeding during laparotomy or abdominal incision). These blood-absorbent wet and cool pads were placed on both sides of the incision while the surgeon continued the operation.

Within a few minutes these pads could be replaced with fresh ones, and anyone would notice that almost all the bleeding had stopped. While occasionally there would be one or two spots that needed to be cauterized, this was very different from the ten to twenty or more spots that were cauterized with the first technique, much less time consuming, with much less injured tissue left behind from the cautery that would cause inflammation and swelling. The second surgeon had taken advantage of the natural clotting ability of the body after trauma. In this case the scalpel was the trauma! And the surgeon was able to quickly continue the procedure.

I saw different techniques in many operations, including how a large surgical wound was repaired at the end of an abdominal surgery, where a thickness of several centimeters on each side of the abdominal incision had to be brought together evenly. Often the surgeon would repair this in layers so that there would be no "dead space," meaning the right side had to fit snugly into the left side without any gaps that could allow a collection of blood, which would be an infection hazard. This meant two suturing repairs. And then there was the excellent surgeon who used a large curved needle to take a generous "bite" of tissue and connect both sides snugly with one suture and there was no dead space. This saved time and the amount of general anesthesia the patient needed. We also saw and enjoyed listening to the singing doctors!

We are taught to limit talking in the operating room because of the danger of microscopic contamination of open wounds by small amounts of saliva, but these doctors faced away from the operative sites as they sang. One Hawaiian doctor, well known for his good voice, was cheered on by the nurses and anyone else close enough to hear him as he would sing an old Hawaiian song in a beautiful loud voice while finishing an operation and suturing the wound.

At another time in Kuakini Hospital, there was an ob-gyn doctor of Japanese descent who would also sing at the end of his operations. This last doctor was also the happiest doctor I have ever met. He was not a youngster but had a wonderful following of patients and was loved by the entire hospital staff. And he had a very nice singing voice. Today this would be considered dangerous!

Chapter Six - Honolulu Dreaming

It was quite a shock to get out of the plane at the Honolulu airport after the nine-hour direct flight from New York City and feel the breezy warm and fragrant air of Hawaii on the island of Oahu and accept the traditional gift of the flower necklace, the lei. I felt wonderful. This was to be where I would work for the next year at the Queen's Hospital in Honolulu and two other hospitals affiliated with the integrated surgical residency program. I definitely experienced "Polynesian paralysis," a feeling of calm and lethargy due to the pleasant, enveloping atmosphere of Hawaii.

My wife and I were very excited to have traveled this far to such a beautiful place and for the opportunity to live here for one year. The surgical residency programs available in New York City did not pay a living wage. All they offered was $4,000 for the year of surgical residency, and we had to take care of our own rental living accommodations in this very high cost city. The Honolulu program, on the other hand, paid $8,000, a living wage in 1968.

We arrived at the height of the summer season, a wonderful time of year in Hawaii. I was to find out that winter in Oahu was the rainy season with modestly cooler temps, but we wouldn't feel that for a long time. We stayed in a low-cost hotel at first until we could find a decent home at a reasonable price and ultimately lived in three different houses in that one year. We were in our mid-twenties and had been married four years.

In two busy weeks, my wife and I would rent a lovely small house in a nice neighborhood about five miles from the hospital. At that same time we also got two used cars, allowing me to commute to the hospital and my wife to go to town for groceries or other things that we needed. This was a very common way for people staying a short period of time in Hawaii to get usable transportation. And those cars did last, with only minor repairs, until we were ready to leave, at which point we sold them for 20 percent less than we had paid for them. People had told us that it was very expensive to live in Hawaii, but we found that if you "went Hawaiian" without duplicating New York City foods, necessities were less expensive than back home.

For example, we had the best fruit at very reasonable prices. We ate delicious ripe pineapples every week and enjoyed mangoes and papayas and bananas. But if we had decided to get apples or peaches or plums from the mainland, they would have been expensive and probably not that fresh. An extra bonus was the fruit trees we had at our rented houses, which had limes and mangoes. We ate local chicken, pork and fish instead of beef, and more rice than bread. We found that Asian restaurants in Honolulu were very reasonably priced with excellent food different from what we were used to in New York City. We had our first taste of Korean food and quite different Chinese food as well as wonderful Japanese food, including our first experiences with sushi and sashimi.

Almost every weekend I had off that summer we could count on beautiful weather and we would go to a beach to swim in the warm water and sunbathe. I even bought a small used sailboat and got a book to teach me how to sail. We had some fun times on that boat, along with one terrifying experience when we neglected to check for any small-craft warnings.

Within a minute or two after launching from the beach that day, we were far out from shore in windy conditions with no other boats around. I was unable to sail the course I wanted back to the beach where we started, and my wife was screaming and crying. Luckily I remembered the old saying "any port in a storm" and set a course to shore a good distance from where we started and made a safe landing. A friendly local beachgoer volunteered to drive us to our car, which was a few miles away. We never did ocean sailing again but still enjoyed the bays and inlets.

New Year's Eve 1969 was amazing.

The interns at the Queen's Hospital planned an outdoor party with live music in a small park. It was a very warm night, so we dressed in summertime clothing, short-sleeve shirts, shorts, short skirts, thin blouses and sandals. Everyone was dancing, and we changed partners as we danced with nurses from the hospital as well as with the interns and residents and their wives or girlfriends.

And then I saw my girlfriend arrive at the party. She was greeted by a lot of people. We all liked her and were happy to see her, but I was a little frightened that my hospital girlfriend and my wife would meet and there would be big problems. My wife wanted to meet this popular girl and I introduced her. Thankfully there was no trouble, that night. We went on to have a wonderful time, and I had a chance to dance with both women I loved on that unforgettable enchanted Hawaiian New Year's Eve.

Chapter Seven - Becoming a Surgeon

Surgeons are not born, they are created. I had come from a medical internship after four years in medical school and I understood how to take a history and do a physical examination and try to decipher what was wrong with the patient. We had plain x-rays, which basically hadn't varied for about fifty years. The wonderful age of CAT scans and MRIs had not yet shown themselves. We didn't even have an ultrasound for diagnosis.

In the first week of my general surgery residency I assisted a senior surgeon performing a hernia repair. When the operation was over, the surgeon asked me to suture the wound and he would be back in fifteen minutes. The scrub nurse handed me the suturing instrument already prepared with a round needle and thin black silk thread. I remembered how to suture from the one time that I sutured a wound that I had made as part of the surgical training course in medical school using anesthetized dogs instead of anesthetized human patients.

I carefully moved the needle through the skin on one side and connected it to the opposite side. I did this a number of times and still found that it wasn't closed properly. so I went back and added a number of sutures on top of the sutures I had already applied. These were separate sutures and I must have had at least fifteen of them with some overlapping until I finally closed the surgical wound. When I was finished and looked at the result, it didn't look exactly the way I thought it should look, but I would wait for the surgeon to return and analyze what I had done.

Within a few minutes the surgeon returned and after looking at the repair I had done, he shook his head and told me this was the worst suturing and closure he had ever seen. And he walked away still shaking his head while the scrub nurse dressed the wound. You can imagine how I felt at that time, and I was determined to quickly improve my surgical skills. When I returned home that evening and for the next few evenings, I used a roll of suture material and practiced the special surgical knots on a bed post until I thought that I was as good as anyone else in tying sutures. I volunteered to suture wounds in the emergency room, and I was lucky to have good attendings to quickly help me escalate my skills dramatically over the next few weeks. This was one of those very exciting times in my education when the amount of improvement and the amount of learning was very high per unit of time compared to other times in high school and college and medical school.

In this residency program I worked primarily in general surgery, which involved abdominal surgery for the most part. This included exploratory surgery when there was no exact diagnosis and the only way to find the problem was to make a large incision in the abdomen, retract the sides, control the bleeding from the incision and explore the different organs of the abdomen, the gallbladder, liver, stomach, spleen and so on. We did this with gloved hands and the touch of our fingers as well as by direct visualization with bright overhead lights. When we found an abnormality we addressed it surgically by removing a tumor or doing a biopsy.

After the operation was over there was a large area to repair and my suturing at this point was complimented by the senior surgeons. In this residency we also had the chance to take electives and my chosen elective was plastic surgery. I already had a residency acceptance in otolaryngology at the New York Eye and Ear Infirmary in New York City, which I would start after I finished this special one-year surgical residency, with a plastic surgery elective. This plastic surgery elective fit perfectly into my upcoming residency. We also did gyn surgery, urological surgery, neurosurgery, vascular surgery, head and neck surgery, eye surgery, ear, nose and throat surgery, and trauma surgery. There was a lot of trauma in Honolulu at that time due to all of the new buildings that were being rapidly constructed.

I remember one case of a middle-aged construction worker falling from a great height and fracturing his skull in several places. He was comatose with multiple open skull wounds, and his brain tissue was exposed with lots of bleeding when he was brought to the operating room. I worked with the neurosurgeon to try to fix any damage that we could, but unfortunately the trauma was too severe and this patient expired on the operating table. The surgeon then gave me a task that I was not trained for. I had to meet with his family and explain that we tried our best and we were very sorry for their loss. I met the tearful wife and the children. It was the eight-year-old boy who got my attention, and I explained that this was the worst injury we had ever seen. Looking at the boy, I said, "Your father was a very strong man to have survived as long as he did after the terrible injuries that he had," and I could see the pride in the boy's tearful face and knew he would always remember and be proud of how strong his father was. This is how we learn to soften the horror of unexpected traumatic death.

In this neurosurgery rotation I also learned what "pulling the plug" meant. I always thought it was a euphemism for ending something, but I learned it had specific meaning in neurosurgery at that time. If we only had five "Bird respirators" for five comatose patients, several of whom had very little chance of survival, and if a new trauma patient in a coma was brought to us, we had to make a difficult decision, and this was the job of the neurosurgeon. That surgeon would choose the patient who was neurologically dead, or "brain dead," already, and a resident who hadn't done it before would unplug the patient from his "Bird," as we called it, after the name of the inventor, and pronounce the patient dead. The new, acutely injured comatose patient would then be placed on the Bird and have an increased chance of survival.

It was interesting to see all of the different techniques that the various surgeons used and to learn new operative skills daily in the operating rooms at the Queen's Hospital, which was run very efficiently. In all of the other experiences I have had with operating rooms I have never seen them run anywhere near as efficiently as this one. Operations started at 7:30 in the morning, but often they would start at 7:15. To start on time, several people had to be present and prepared at the same time: the anesthesiologist, if the surgery was under general anesthesia, the scrub nurse, the circulating nurse, the surgeon, surgical assistant, and of course, the patient.

In every other hospital I've worked at there would usually be at least one of those important people who would be late, which would obviously delay surgery. This would also delay everything else in the surgeon's schedule and the use of the operating rooms.

Gradually I became a surgeon, and by the end of that year I felt very confident in my skills involving scalpels, retractors, lighting and suturing as well as interacting with all the other personnel. There are several things surgeons need to be superior in their performance. I think good vision is the most important element, and after that comes hand skills. I knew a young doctor who wanted to become an expert at microsurgery, but he was excluded from the specialty program because he had large hands. This was an error on the part of the senior surgeon who turned him down, because although it seems that we operate with our hands, we really operate with the instruments that we hold in our fingers in microsurgery.

Most doctors take academic courses in their pre-medical school education. When you think about it, we spend many years through grade school, high school and college where we will learn calculus, foreign languages and other intellectual studies, but we neglect to be taught hand skills such as assembling things, taking things apart, reconstructing, carving, sewing, drawing and so on. I found it ironic that the first time I ever used a hand drill was in my neurosurgery training on a patient's head to drain a life-threatening subdural hematoma. I didn't expect the neurosurgeon to give me the hand drill and show me the four marked spaces on the shaved skull where I was to drill a hole. As I started drilling I asked the surgeon how I would know that I had gone far enough and not too far. He laughed a little and said, "You'll know," and he and the anesthesiologist both laughed. I made all the drill holes and was complimented on my technique.

In the days before safe and effective anesthesia, surgeons had to be experts in anatomy and in the ability to operate quickly. Today we're lucky to have both the anatomy skills and the ability to operate at a more reasonable pace because of excellent anesthesia. Stamina is another requirement for surgeons, since an operation can take much longer than planned due to unexpected findings or mishaps in the operating room.

We also need the ability to stand or sit for long periods of time without a continuous need for bathroom breaks or food and water breaks. Several times in my operating career I had to stand and assist at the side of the operating table for as long as twelve consecutive hours. Luckily this was not common. In my career as an ear, nose and throat doctor, most of the surgeries that I performed were less than two hours, although some of the operations could be as long as three to four hours. A good surgeon must be able to keep the operation going smoothly without delays or repeating the moves, such as making an additional incision instead of getting the original incision right. I've had the opportunity over the years to watch many surgeons operate, and sometimes I had to leave the operating room, unable to watch a surgeon because of the poor surgical technique. At other times I learned how to improve my technique by watching superior surgeons.

Unfortunately, even the best surgeon has a finite career of excellent performance. I watched many senior surgeons operating into their seventies and noted changes in their abilities. Even though they were still competent, they were not the same. I guess all physical performers experience this. It's sad to watch the once great boxer or baseball or basketball player perform past his prime, and surgery is no different. Oh, there's one last requirement to be a great surgeon, and that is to know when NOT to operate, since there are often medical treatments and lifestyle changes that can solve the problem, or the patient may not be a good candidate for a particular surgery.

Chapter Eight - Brooklyn Meets Alabama

I never expected to have a friend from Alabama. My upbringing in Brooklyn didn't include anyone from the South, and this was a time in American history when the South was in turmoil. I recall black and white images on our family's TV showing federally enforced integration of schools and communities, swelling civil rights marches and disturbing scenes of riots and attack dogs used to intimidate "colored people" and prevent them from enjoying the same rights and privileges that I had in America.

Several of the prominent surgeons who I worked with at the Queen's Hospital in Honolulu in 1968 were from the South. It was my first exposure to people who grew up below the Mason-Dixon line, something I'd heard about only in American Civil War history. After working shoulder to shoulder with them, I realized that these were great surgeons, and on an individual basis they did not show prejudice or racism against people of color.

As a surgical resident, one senior doctor stands out in my mind, and that was Dr. Robert Flowers. He was a youthful attending plastic surgeon who befriended me. I was the only East Coast doctor in the program, which made me the exotic young doctor from New York City. He taught me plastic surgery techniques that were invaluable to me during my surgical career and told me stories about his surgical residency, where he was required to watch many surgeries before he was allowed to do any part of the surgery. This was in contrast to my experience in New York City, where the surgeons in training would be eager to cut and explore very early in their careers. In fact I had thought that early performance of surgical procedures by interns and residents was the key to proficiency. In the plastic surgery elective I took during my general surgery training, I had many opportunities to watch and assist Dr. Flowers, and he taught me things I had never imagined were important.

One morning I was assisting him on a face lift and he pointed out that I was gripping the facial tissue too firmly with my forceps. He explained why the gentlest pressure was all that was needed. Otherwise I might be leaving injured tissue behind, which could increase postoperative swelling, redness and pain, and possibly lead to infection. And sure enough, when I loosened my grip, I noticed that the skin was indented with slight bruising.

After working with Dr. Flowers for a few months and learning so many things, I was surprised one day when he asked if I would like to join his plastic surgery practice. He said I already had acquired many plastic surgical skills and he was impressed with my overall surgical abilities, keen eyesight, steady hands and dexterity. I was very flattered by this offer. He said I wouldn't need a whole plastic surgery residency, just one more year of general surgery and then I would work with him, and in that way I would earn plastic surgery certification since he was one of the examiners for the board of plastic surgery. I thanked him again for all he had taught me. But I explained I was very interested in the new field of microsurgery in ENT, and I had already accepted a residency in New York City at the New York Eye and Ear Infirmary and I would still be able to use my newly acquired plastic surgery skills to do facial plastic surgery for much of my career. I have lived through plenty of frigid Northeastern winters since I rejected that generous offer from Dr. Flowers, and sometimes I daydream about the life I would have had if I had said yes.

Dr. Flowers and I also had opportunities to talk politics. He said it was past time to get rid of the old segregation habit, the Jim Crow laws in the South, and he was embarrassed at all the attempts to maintain them and the ugly displays of Southern racism portrayed on TV at this time. He was surprised when I told him about the all-white neighborhoods I grew up in when I was raised in Brooklyn in the 1940s and 1950s. He said he guessed the North and South were not as different as he had thought, but that the North had certainly advanced more over time than the South.

One day Dr. Flowers came up to me all excited to tell me that we had the worst-behaved patient anyone could ever have on our surgical floor. I remember him saying in his Southern accent that we had an arrogant New Yorker who didn't think we knew anything about plastic surgery and was continually on the phone with his New York doctors checking every step of the complicated treatment and repair of his ankle injury he got while playing golf. Apparently his golf cart skidded off the path and scraped the skin off his medial malleolus, which is an area of the ankle very difficult to skin graft successfully.

At first I was taken aback by the negative reference to New York since I was a proud New Yorker, living in New York City for years and having a three-year specialty residency there coming up after finishing this surgical residency.

Obviously this frightened patient, far out of his comfort zone, didn't know that he had one of the very best plastic surgeons anywhere in the United States helping him. I realize that many people may have thought that Hawaii was just a big vacation resort. How could there be great surgeons outside of New York City or any other big city with large teaching hospitals, and what was the possibility of such surgeons existing in the remote islands of Hawaii? In fact, this may be the reason that the Queen's Hospital and the Honolulu integrated surgical residency had a hard time filling their resident positions and that was why I was the only resident who came from New York City.

Dr. Flowers wanted me to see this difficult patient. When I first glimpsed him while I was still out of his room, he was propped up on his hospital bed with the phone to his ear shouting questions about the treatment he was getting to his doctors back in New York City. This was decades before the time of cell phones, but this patient demanded and received a scarce house phone on his night table around the clock.

The nurses were warning me about encountering this patient. They said that he was the worst-behaved patient they had ever seen. He was terrible and mean to them with never a kind word or thank you for all the things they did for him. I quickly saw and heard this frightened patient talking down to his doctors and yelling at the nurses, as he continuously complained about one thing or another. He even berated the excellent plastic surgeon Dr. Flowers, who was able to control himself and act professionally at all times. I thought about entering his room and trying to calm him down, but I was the plastic surgery resident and I was already late for a major nasal reconstruction after an automobile accident.

I felt sad for this man who was definitely not a typical New Yorker, and I hoped he would ultimately be appreciative of the excellent care he was getting and would apologize for any rudeness he had displayed.

Chapter Nine - HIV

In the early 1980s, doctors started to notice and talk about a new lethal disease affecting young people. They were getting rare infections and tumors and invariably died of this disease even with the best medical care. This new disease was mostly affecting the gay community and intravenous drug users. A common thread of this disease was announced by the CDC and turned into the "four H's"—homosexuality, heroin, hemophilia and Haitian—to help doctors diagnose this new disease.

We didn't know what the presumed organism was that caused this, and we also heard that doctors got this fatal disease from blood contact with ill victims, from accidental needle sticks after taking blood from a sick patient or from operating on those who had this mystery disease. A new epidemic was unfolding in front of doctors, health care workers and the general public. Famous people were getting this new disease, and this was interesting news to report. The CDC was working hard to identify an organism so that people could be tested for it and a possible cure could be developed. Patients didn't survive once they had the disease. Curiously, patients did not have to tell doctors that they were infected when they sought care, but doctors who were infected had to tell their patients.

This epidemic started with a small number of cases. In the old days of treating epidemics or venereal diseases, a person infected would be interviewed to discover any contacts that could become sick or who could spread the disease, but this "plague" was different. There were no quarantines, one of the oldest techniques to control an epidemic. Just the reverse was employed, where the patients could be anonymous and unintentionally spread the illness widely. I remember talking to other doctors to get their opinion as to the causative agent.

A gastroenterologist suggested that this might be a reaction to semen implanted during anal intercourse. Another doctor who was very religious thought it was God's punishment for homosexuality. But, like most doctors, I thought it was a viral disease.

Luckily, fastidious researchers were able to find the virus that they called "human immunodeficiency virus" (HIV), and then tests were devised for detecting "acquired immunodeficiency syndrome" or "AIDS," as it was commonly called. Several antiviral drugs were tested, and finally excellent, effective treatments were available although only for controlling the virus and not for curing it. Infected patients needed to take the medicine all the time or the disease would return with deadly consequences. This was a triumph of rapid medical research and pharmaceutical production.

Unfortunately, poorer countries dealing with this infection had to pay the prevailing U.S. cost of the patented medication, which was in the range of thousands of dollars per month. When India needed the medication for tens of thousands of patients, they wisely "broke" the patent held by U.S pharmaceutical companies, with apologies, and produced the medications at a very small fraction of the patented cost, and thus were now able to treat their sick AIDS population.

To this day I feel that the epidemic might have been controlled with the old techniques of quarantine and patient interviews with contact follow-ups. I remember seeing pictures of homes with quarantine signs from the department of health when I was a youngster. Violation of the quarantine by leaving your home or having unauthorized visitors was a crime for which you could be fined and possibly vulnerable to prison time.

Chapter Ten - The Party's Over

1969 in Honolulu

I was turning into a surgeon with the help of the wonderful surgical residency I was taking, and I was also having the time of my young life with the experience of living in Hawaii with my wife, and spending time with my girlfriend at the Queen's Hospital, a very common arrangement at the hospital where I worked. My wife enjoyed being with me in Hawaii, in a series of comfortable houses, and the wonderful activities we had together when I was off from my hospital duties. And I had a lovely girlfriend at the hospital who looked forward, as I did, to our times together. I knew I was "cheating" on my wife but it didn't seem to be such a big deal to me at this time since the practice was so common, especially in the era of the '60s, and I did spend much more time with my wife than with my girlfriend.

Historically, powerful men had more than one wife, and maybe that was natural, and it certainly felt natural to me as strange as it sounds. On the weekends my wife and I would go to one of many beaches we liked, and we would dine out in Honolulu at wonderful restaurants and even host friends at our house. We had an active sex life together, although we had to be careful about unwanted pregnancy since my wife did not want to have a baby at this time, so we were careful with a diaphragm and monitoring her cycles. With my girlfriend I had to be extremely careful to not have a pregnancy even though she was taking birth control pills.

I met my girlfriend in her private office on the hospital campus, and at times when I was taking call. And sometimes when I told my wife I was staying late at the hospital or going to the evening art class at Honolulu University, where I was taking a course on painting with acrylics with an intern friend of mine. This arrangement lasted for a long time and seemed to work for me and the two women. My girlfriend knew that our relationship would only last until I needed to go back to New York City with my wife, and this was the case with many other interns and residents who had one-year contracts at the hospital. I also had the impression that the hospital staff interested in these exciting affairs would have new partners when next year's interns and residents appeared.

Then one night when I had told my wife that I would be late, I overstayed the lateness with my girlfriend. When I realized the time, I quickly said goodbye to her and raced back home. I was met by an unsmiling wife at the door and knew immediately that she had found out about the secret arrangement. "Where were you?" she tearily demanded to know. "I called the Queen's Hospital and there was no meeting that night, and I called Kuakini Hospital, and the hospital operator said there was no meeting there. I could hear her friend laughing when I said, 'Where could he be?' He told me there was a meeting and the other hospitals said there was no meeting."

I told her that I was seeing a girl at the hospital, and she broke down and collapsed with heart-wrenching sobbing. She wasn't able to yell at me, just loud sobbing and crying, and I hugged her and we sat down and I said I was so sorry. She cried and sobbed most of the night. Finally toward morning she was able to ask how long had this been going on and I said a few months and the crying and sobbing came back again. I comforted her as much as I could and made some tea and gave it to her with buttered bread and told her I loved her and I was so sorry for what I had done and I would never do that again. She made me promise I would never see or talk to this girl again or contact her in any way, and I said I would do that and I told her I had to leave for the hospital. I hugged her again and left the house with a great sadness for the grief I caused her.

As I approached the hospital, I stopped to call my girlfriend and tell her it was over, that my wife had called all the hospitals before I came home so late, and no one knew where I was, and I had to tell her about us and she collapsed and broke down.

I said I wouldn't be meeting her for breakfast anymore, and she started crying and asked, "Will we never see each other again?" And I said, "Yes," and the crying was louder with choking and gagging as she said, "Please, just let me see you one more time." And I told her, "I promised my wife that I wouldn't even call you, and I can't see you again." She couldn't speak and could barely breathe and I heard her choking again and I told her I was so sorry and I would call her later and she said she couldn't go to work so I could call her anytime, and we said goodbye.

When I called her at lunchtime she said she felt sick and couldn't eat anything.

She always knew that our relationship would be over at the end of the residency, and she was prepared for that, but not for this sudden ending, and she started crying again and begged me to see her one more time so we could really say goodbye. I said I couldn't, and she kept crying and I told her I loved her and I will always love the time we had together and I could never forget her, but we couldn't see each other again, and I said I was so sorry to hurt her. She continued crying and I told her, "I'm sorry but I have to go to surgery now." I felt terrible that I had hurt the two women I loved. I guess I never thought this would happen so suddenly and painfully for all three of us. I always thought the affair would end peacefully, as planned, at the end of my residency.

By the time my wife and I returned to New York City we had discussed the possibility of an "open marriage," where we each could have short extramarital affairs without cheating and still love each other. This was being promoted during the accelerated sexual revolution of the '60s, and we considered this not long after our return to New York City.

Chapter Eleven - My Otolaryngology Residency

My general surgery residency ended on the last day of June, and my ENT (ear, nose and throat) residency began on the first day of July. Since I had to travel thousands of miles from Honolulu to get to my new residency in New York City, it was difficult for me to start on July first, and I missed the first day of the new residency and was harshly criticized for this.

Once again I was considered to be the exotic doctor because I had gone to Hawaii for my training in general surgery rather than taking it in the important and famous New York City hospitals that almost everyone else had done. Every doctor I met had the impression that the residency in the faraway hospitals in Honolulu could not have been that good since Honolulu was a vacation destination.

The first days, weeks and months of this three-year specialty residency program at the New York Eye and Ear Infirmary were as exciting as the first few weeks and months of the general surgery residency that I had just completed. Once again I was learning new things at a very rapid pace and enjoying every hour of this training program. Fortunately we had an excellent young ear, nose and throat attending doctor as the director of the clinic teaching program, and I was able to verify with him the things that I saw and heard while examining the patients in the clinic before I prescribed medication or recommended treatment.

Basically, we were learning three specialties at the same time, since examination of the ears is quite different from examination of the nose or throat and required different instruments and techniques, making this a thrilling learning adventure for me. We also had to master the head mirror worn on our forehead that focused a beam of light from a lamp behind the patient's head and allowed us to see deep into the throat or nose or ear. The head mirror became another part of our bodies after a while, so that we barely felt it on our heads and I sometimes had to be reminded to take it off when I had left the clinic. We took a history and examined the patient with only a thin curtain separating us from the other residents who were doing the same thing right next to us.

This was an era when the concept of complete privacy, visual and auditory, for an examination that did not involve removing shirts or pants or skirts had not been mandated, and this allowed us to have easy access to the program director and other attending doctors when we needed help with the patient rather than having to open a door and travel, even if only a few steps, to see and talk privately to the experienced doctors.

There were fifteen resident doctors in this training program, five in each of the three years, and all of the first-year residents, including myself, had to be available in clinic at one o'clock sharp for the start of the afternoon clinic. Two of the second-year residents and one of the senior-year residents also worked in this afternoon clinic. We saw many patients every day, some with so-called minor problems, such as excess earwax, or major problems, such as facial paralysis or loss of voice or bleeding from the nose, as well as problems that were not as common but very troublesome to the patients like TMJ syndrome, with ear and jaw joint pain upon opening the mouth wide. We had lectures from dental surgeons on this last problem and noted it was predominantly young women suffering from it. We suspected it was from the increasing popularity of oral sex, especially after the blockbuster movie *Deep Throat*, although many dentists blamed TMJ on dental malocclusion and bruxism (grinding of teeth) and thought the solution was dental braces.

We addressed all of these problems, gave advice and often did the treatments at the same time as well as prescribing medication and further testing and follow-up as needed. Sometimes surgery would be recommended. In this way we were able to treat fifty to one hundred patients or more until the end of the clinic at four o'clock, or later if needed.

Eight doctors were in the clinic every weekday, and there was a smaller clinic on Saturday morning with only first-year residents plus availability to see patients at any time day or night if there was a serious emergency. This was considered a walk-in clinic without the need for an appointment to be seen as long as you arrived before 3 P.M., and this was probably the way the clinic had been run since its inception in the 1800s, when this unique specialty hospital was founded with a grant from New York State.

Some very old doctors at the hospital told me that there used to be a large bowl at the entrance to the clinic, and as the patients entered the clinic they put a quarter into the bowl, and before that, it used to be a dime. A major learning advantage in this clinic was that follow-up visits to check the progress of the original illness and treatment were always taken care of by the doctor who saw the patient the first time. This was similar to how a private doctor would follow-up his patients at this time before group practice became common. We also had an allergy clinic once a week in the morning and we rotated our coverage of this clinic with the other first-year residents as we worked with a senior allergy doctor and nurses who mixed the allergy shots.

Our surgical experience as first-year residents consisted of tonsillectomy and adenoidectomy, as well as nasal surgery like "SMR," which was short for "submucous resection," to correct septal deviations, which inhibited good nasal breathing. We also did nasal polypectomy, which involved snaring and removal of benign obstructive nasal polyps. We were all surgeons at this point and licensed by New York State. We learned these operations from senior residents and attending doctors. But the time came when we had to do these operations by ourselves.

We were surprised to learn that we had to do these operations in the nose by ourselves as the only trained medical person in the operating room with the patient. We did have a heavy brass bell that we could ring if we needed help from a circulating nurse or other medical personnel. I often thought that these were the original bells used in the 1800s. The operating room lighting was purposely dim, and we had battery-operated headlights, which illuminated the areas that we needed to see.

All the instruments and all of the medications for numbing the nose were on a small table adjacent to the operating bed. For nasal operations we used topical cocaine and injectable local anesthetics with all the needles and syringes necessary for injecting lidocaine, also known as Xylocaine. Patients reclined on the back of the operating table awake so that they could change position as needed. Any bleeding could be removed with a gauze pad or a suction tube.

Once the topical and injectable anesthetics had taken effect, there was no pain for the patient, although anxiety and fear persisted, and it was important to keep talking to patients to reassure them that everything was going well and the operation would shortly be over. These two operations, one on the nasal septum and the other on nasal polyps, usually were completed within thirty minutes, and then gauze packing was inserted into the nose to prevent excess bleeding, and the patient was helped off the table and to the recovery area.

I found these operations to be fairly simple since I had seen them and assisted on these cases while working with ENT doctors in Honolulu, but my first-year colleagues often had great difficulty with them. I remember one time I was called into an adjacent operating room by one of my colleagues because he had lost his orientation inside the nose of a patient he was operating on for deviated septum. I wanted to help him but looking into the nose from the side all I could see was blood clots. I would have had to stop his operation, and mine, and do his by myself to correct any problems, and that would be very irregular and could get both of us into a lot of trouble. I told him it was time to ring the big brass bell.

A much more difficult operation to be done solo was the adult tonsillectomy.

Most adult tonsillectomies, just like children's tonsillectomies, were performed in the operating room with general anesthesia, but there was a history of doing many operations under local anesthesia dating back to a time when general anesthesia was risky, which is quite different today. And even in 1969 when I did these cases, there were still situations where a local anesthetic would be safer.

Once again we were alone doing this more complex operation with a patient who was awake. To make this even more interesting, the patient was the one who had to hold his tongue down with a curved metal retractor so that we could have both hands free to operate on the tonsils in the back of the throat on each side. We used topical and injectable local anesthetics so that the patient would feel no pain from the surgery.

One advantage of the local tonsillectomy was that the injectable anesthetic also had a vasoconstrictor, which limited the bleeding during surgery that had to be suctioned out of the throat. In any event this was a stressful operation for the patient and the doctor.

Some people in the hospital were starting to think that the local tonsillectomy was an outdated operation. Within a short period of time, one of the scrub nurses volunteered to assist me during these operations so that the patients did not have to hold their own retractor and the surgeon would not have to also do the suctioning of blood as the operation proceeded. Not many more local tonsillectomies were performed after my residency.

The second-year residents were taught sinus surgery, laryngoscopy, bronchoscopy and esophagoscopy. The senior or third-year residents, who would be graduating that year, were taught head and neck surgery and ear surgery, including middle ear microsurgery and facial plastic surgery. This teaching hierarchy was strictly enforced, so that even though I had assisted on many plastic surgery operations in Honolulu, I was unable to do these surgeries until my senior year.

Nevertheless I was able to "sneak" in a minor rhinoplasty on a sinus patient with a difficult deviated septum while I was a second-year resident by performing a shortening of a long nose at the same time, with only minor criticism from my superiors since there were no complications and the patient was very happy with the results.

There was a time when senior residents competed for the title of chief resident, but by the time I was a senior resident, all senior residents were considered chief residents and there was less stress as we completed our training. I learned from older surgeons that there was a great advantage to being "the chief" in the previous era and that each resident would work as many hours as possible to earn that distinction. One retired surgeon in Honolulu told me he was so exhausted and "wound up" after working more than forty-eight hours straight without a break that when he got home he would drink liquor until he passed out. And he became an alcoholic.

Luckily in my training there were more surgeons and no need for marathon workloads or the stress of competing against our resident friends. We even had time off during the day where we could study or watch an expert surgeon operate, and we also had a full hour for lunch every day! but, like every other resident, we periodically had the annoying "on call" responsibility.

Sadly at this time my wife and I were having marital problems. Our marriage had suffered from my affair in Honolulu and then improved but was ultimately destroyed by the influence of the accelerated sexual revolution in New York City at that time when women were wearing see-through blouses, and casual affairs and wife swapping were common. We drifted apart and then divorced during my ENT residency.

Otolaryngology was undergoing major changes and challenges in this time period, expanding head and neck procedures to include radical cancer operations, thyroid operations and more facial plastic surgeries. Our specialty was encroaching on established head and neck surgeons, plastic surgeons and thyroid surgeons. There were even lawsuits brought against our medical societies to prevent what must have felt like illegal trespassing or stealing to these other specialists. Unfortunately at this same time we neglected to continue our long surgical tradition of diagnostic bronchoscopy and esophagoscopy. These areas were taken over by internal medicine specialists, and we were only called in for difficult foreign body removal cases.

At my interview with the chief of surgery for hospital privileges at the start of my first solo private practice as a certified ENT specialist, I was told, in a loud voice by the physically impressive chief of surgery: "You will not do thyroid surgery at this hospital." There was no discussion after he told me this. This was not too important to me because, as a newly trained specialist with proficiency in many operations and opening up a practice in a community with a shortage of ENT specialists, I was bound to be busy enough without thyroid surgery.

I actually had my first private patient in my office before its construction was finished. One of the workers building the office had a clogged ear, and my examination showed the common malady of impacted cerumen, an ear clogged with wax, and I was quickly able to cure him with the excellent German-made stainless-steel syringe that many ENT doctors in this era had in their bag of instruments. He was very happy with the improved hearing. I charged him fifteen dollars and that doubled the money I had in my pocket.

Chapter Twelve - On Call

Once you get the MD or other practitioner degree and work at a hospital, you will become part of the "on call" world. Doctors need sleep as much as anyone else and should be entitled to a good sleep most nights. In order for this to happen there has to be at least one doctor "on call" to take care of emergencies at night when all the regular support staff has left the hospital. The on-call doc may lose a night's sleep, but all the other docs get to sleep. On call usually starts late afternoon and runs until the following morning. Depending on the number of doctors to share this chore, the "call" could be once a week or several weeks or variations of that.

Hospitals are busy places in the daytime, with large numbers of doctors, nurses and ancillary staff, including secretaries, PAs (physician assistants), NPs (nurse practitioners), medical students, visitors, administrators and so on. The hospital seems to be in motion as if someone wound up a large toy or carousel. Noise levels are high and people move quickly from one duty to another, including visits to cafeterias and restrooms.

And then it all stops!

The lighting dims, the place of such hustle and bustle just minutes before turns into a slow-motion, quiet experience. Then loneliness starts. The on-call doctor is away from family and friends, isolated. My worst on-call experiences were on Thanksgiving, my favorite holiday, with feasting and fun time with favorite relatives. There's always an on-call room with a bed for the docs, and this may be a shared room with several other on-call docs, or a private room, or it may be more elaborate with a second room, a toilet and a shower.

As the night progresses, loneliness may increase. But there are other lonely people in the hospital, too, and sometimes two lonely people can meet and dispel the loneliness. Doctors and nurses have long been associated with each other, and often date or marry. Mononucleosis, often called "mono" is a common contagious viral disease associated with kissing, and it used to be called the doctors and nurses' disease, a possible reference to intimate friendliness of the two professions, at least in the past.

And so it might have occurred that a lonely doctor and a lonely nurse with access to a private room were able to pass a pleasant and stimulating evening with romance, and chase the loneliness away. Thus an onerous assignment could turn into one that might be sought after as long as there weren't too many emergencies.

One of the interns at the Queen's Hospital in Honolulu was always "busy" on the nights when he "took call." In a reversal from the old story of the ship's captain with a girl in every port, this intern was a frequent partner of a stewardess who had a "lover" in every airport!

One summer night when my wife and I were newly separated and I was taking call, I looked out a hospital window and saw a party going on in a building across the street and this got me even more depressed with the on-call night and my marital sadness.

I started walking the halls of the hospital to take my mind off my predicament and I ran into the pretty nurse who had helped me with the adult tonsillectomy under local anesthesia, and I was surprised to see her this late in the hospital. I said "hi," and she stopped as she recognized me. I asked her what she was doing in the hospital so late. Was there an emergency operation I should know about? She smiled and said she lived in the hospital.

I thought she was joking, but she told me she lived in the old wing of the hospital, which I had never seen. I asked her where it was, and she said she would show me. We walked to a part of the hospital I didn't know existed, and there was a long line of clean white sheet-covered hospital beds, as if they were silently waiting for an influx of patients. We walked past these beds until we got to one that looked used, with clothing on an adjacent bed. She said the hospital allows full-time medical employees to live there free of charge, but this was temporary since she was looking for a small apartment in the neighborhood.

We sat on the bed and chatted. At one point she said she was chilled and I moved closer and put my arm around her. She leaned against me, and then we kissed, and things got a lot more exciting over the next hour. That was the start of our relationship, which ended without tears when I graduated from the residency and left New York City to begin my first full-time specialty practice. Shortly thereafter I met the woman who would be my second wife and the mother of our children and the grandma of our grandchildren.

Footnote: The above was experienced in an era when there were no cell phones or electronic social media to keep isolated people in touch with their friends and families. Many things that were accepted in this era would definitely not be acceptable today. Also at this time most doctors and almost all surgeons were male and almost all nurses were female.

An additional footnote: This old hospital area, called the "ghost hospital" by some, was also the setting for the scene in *The Godfather* where Marlon Brando was lying on one of those old ghost hospital beds.

Chapter Thirteen - Moonlighting

In the 1960s and '70s the hospitals with internship and residency programs were gradually increasing salaries of the "house officers," as we were known, but the salaries relative to hours of work were still pitiful, and most docs were unable to live on these wages. A working spouse was a big help, and most of the docs I worked with were married in their twenties and getting support from spouse or parents, but this was still not enough, especially if small children were involved, thus "moonlighting"—the term applied to night work or other work to generate extra income.

Most hospitals decried this activity but would usually wink at it, and in some cases there were established relationships between hospitals' doctors and a "moonlighting" facility. The New York Eye and Ear Infirmary had a relationship with the Rikers Island prison, and brave residents would spend a night there taking care of any medical problems the inmates or any prison staff might have while earning a salary.

These doctors, as you might imagine, lost a good night's sleep, and the other residents would cover for them and let them sleep in the on-call rooms or the "ghost" hospital, also called the "old" hospital, at the New York Eye and Ear, which still had dozens of hospital beds carefully maintained by the housekeeping personnel. We let them sleep till noon when once again they would be fit for regular hospital duties.

I didn't like the idea of a night shift at a prison, so I had to construct my own moonlighting career, and I did it piecemeal. I had an uncle who sold life insurance policies and he would call me in to do the physical exams and certify the insurance seekers as healthy without serious medical conditions. This involved a questionnaire, blood pressure testing and listening to the heart and lungs with a stethoscope, all activities that recent medical graduates were adept at. This activity was sporadic for me, but the fee from the insurance company was at least 20 percent of my weekly salary and sometimes there would be two or three clients to examine at the same time.

In addition I would cover the office practice of various private doctors when they were away on vacation, or out of their office for any other reason, and earn considerably more while practicing my specialty and learning how to treat patients of a different socioeconomic class than the clinic patients we managed at the hospital. On those occasions, when my hospital duties ended, I would dash to the private office and work three or four hours with the secretary, evaluating and treating the private doctor's patients and I would often earn the equivalent of a full week's salary in just two sessions. On another occasion, while I was walking home from my hospital work, I noticed a new dental facility just three blocks from the hospital.

With the new Medicaid laws, there was an unfulfilled demand for dental care among the less affluent, who qualified for this new social program that President Johnson promoted alongside Medicare. This was reminiscent of Franklin Roosevelt's New Deal which gave us Social Security during the Great Depression. I was curious if the director of the dental clinic might have a need for a medical doctor to evaluate patients before extensive dental work.

When I entered the new facility I was greeted by a receptionist and I asked her if I could talk to the director, who promptly appeared. I asked him if he might need a medical doctor, and he immediately asked me if I would like to be the "medical director" of the dental clinic. I said "sure," and that was a position I held for a year until the clinic had to close due to Medicaid investigations over questionable billing for dental procedures. But that was a very interesting and enlightening job for me, and I learned about billing for Medicaid and "factoring," where I would submit my bills to a third party and immediately get 90 percent of the billing. I requested basic instrumentation, including an electrocardiogram machine and some minor surgical tools.

At least twice a week I would walk the three blocks from the hospital to my new office and examine new patients and do cardiograms on the older patients as well as listen to their hearts and lungs and take blood pressures.

I enjoyed working with these new patients and I was able to double my salary, which made paying my bills easier but also taught me more about paying taxes.

The closest I got to having a true general private practice of my own early in my residency was when I saw patients in a small house I shared with my wife in upstate New York.

Her family gave us the down payment on this converted one-room schoolhouse, and we paid the mortgage bill and the upkeep of the house and grounds.

As we got to know people in this community and they found out I was a doctor, some friends asked if I would see them as patients. They wanted a young doctor with progressive thoughts about treatments, including alternatives to the usual testing and antibiotics. And this way I had a general practice on Saturday mornings from 9 A.M. to noon or even later if there were more patients. I treated the usual mix of general practice in mostly young and alternative-culture patients. This era of the hippies had a saying, "Don't trust anyone over 30," and I was under thirty at that time.

The strangest patient I had arrived two hours late and he had walked from town, a distance of several miles, barefoot. His problem was foot pain and bleeding feet. I examined him and saw that he had abrasions of his feet with some bleeding and crusted blood. I got a basin of warm water and some soap and a towel and knelt in front of him and washed his feet. There was no sign of infection or laceration. I got him a pair of socks from my supply of socks and drove him back to his home. I advised him to wear sandals when he went walking in the future. He told me he had no money to pay for the visit and I told him it was all right. What I did for this young man felt biblical.

I never thought I would have an obstetrical practice alongside the private practice upstate, but soon, liberated young pregnant women showed up on my Saturday hours in the old schoolhouse. These were intelligent women who had read about how deliveries were done before the days of hospital care with delivery on your back under sedation. They knew that birthing was always done in a squatting posture helped by women with lots of experience in attending births. They also objected to all the medications that were given to women in labor so that they would not feel any of the pain of childbirth.

These women wanted to "experience" childbirth and not be sedated when their baby was born so that they could immediately hold and bond with their newborn. Some of the women spoke of a "Birth Orgasm" at the moment of delivery. I definitely understood what they wanted and felt that I would want that, too, if I were a woman. But they had to know that since I was a full-time surgical resident, their labor might be in the middle of an operation I was doing and I might not be able to attend to them. I also explained that certain abnormalities might create a risk for them and their baby and that statistically hospital birth might be safer. These women were strong and wanted it their way and would have their babies alone if no one was available to help them. There were no doctors doing what they wanted, and they told me there were no midwives available either. I felt it was my duty to give them at least my obstetrical experience rather than let them try to give birth alone.

I did regular prenatal checkups on the pregnant women as I had been taught in med school, including examining the abdomen to determine the position of the fetus and one cervical evaluation as they got close to the due date. Naturally some of the women dropped out before childbirth due to strong parental objection or from things they heard from friends, but in the end there were two women who persevered and whose active labor and my schedule synced.

Chapter Fourteen - Childbirth

What does an ear, nose and throat doctor know about childbirth?

I went to medical school for four years. I was a medical intern for one year, a surgical resident for one year and finally an otolaryngology resident for three years. My medical license permits me to practice medicine and surgery as a general practitioner. I never lost my interest in general medicine or the history and biology and science that underpins modern medicine.

I was originally attracted to ob-gyn as a specialty but at that time it was all solo practice, being on call for deliveries day and night, and that did not appeal to me. My extensive medical school experience in ob-gyn with sleepless nights turned me from this field. How was I to know that within a few years that stressful ob-gyn routine would turn into group practice with well-defined schedules for the doctors! But I never forgot my extensive obstetrical experiences in medical school with the fifty deliveries I performed. Helping to bring a life into the world was so different from treating sickness and dealing with death. But there were things that troubled me from those hospital deliveries that were still in my mind, and I would find myself thinking about them at times, trying to figure them out.

For example, after the delivery of the newborn, there was a great rush to clamp and then cut the umbilical cord. I was surprised at how difficult it was to clamp that turgid, pumping cord, and this is from a young man not far from the days when he weight-lifted loaded barbells and still had a very strong grip. After the cord was clamped and cut, the baby was handed to a nurse who rushed the infant to a separate area to be analyzed for the Apgar score, which measured how strong and healthy the baby was immediately after delivery. The

Apgar score came from a pediatric anesthesiologist named Virginia Apgar and stands for appearance, pulse, grimace, activity and, finally, respiration.

If a newborn did not get the normal score then the pediatrician would start various treatments to improve the newborn's chance of healthy survival. I wondered why so many newborns were in medical danger so soon after their birth. But when I was working in obstetrics, I did not have time to even walk over to talk with the pediatrician who was assessing the health of the newborn because there was an immediate urgent need to get the placenta delivered. The placenta is commonly called the "afterbirth" since it would be delivered after the birth of the infant.

The crisis we had to deal with at this moment was to get the placenta delivered as quickly as possible, which involved putting large amounts of pressure on the mother's abdomen to push the placenta out of the uterus without leaving any fragments behind. Fragments could cause serious bleeding or lead to infection that might necessitate a hysterectomy. You can imagine how uncomfortable and painful strong pressure applications to the mother's abdomen were right after the struggle of delivery. Often a slim nurse would actually climb onto the mother's abdomen to push even harder. At last the placenta was delivered, albeit with much bleeding due to two factors: the premature clamping of the umbilical cord while it was still delivering blood to the baby, and the violent tearing of the placenta from its uterine attachments caused by the extreme pressure applied to the abdomen.

If there was a chance that some parts of the placenta were not delivered, then the obstetrician would need to do a wiping of the uterus with a gauze pad at the end of a large forceps which caused even more discomfort to the young mother who had just gone through labor and delivery.

I knew from my studies of biology that almost all species of mammals are placental, so that, as in humans, they support the developing animal with nutrients and oxygen through an umbilical cord. It is hard to imagine that any other mammal, for example a horse, a cow, a dog or a cat, would turn around during birthing to bite and sever the umbilical cord while it was still delivering essential blood to its progeny.

Why were humans different? Was there some medical advantage to depriving the newborn of all the blood from the mother through the umbilical cord?

This was what I would ponder at various times.

And then there was the time I had a delivery experience with a private obstetrician in Brooklyn. The attending doctor wanted to further our education and would let us medical students deliver the babies of his private patients without the permission or knowledge of the patient, something that sounds unbelievable in the present era but was considered to be normal teaching in that era. The patient would have sedation and possibly a spinal anesthesia, then a blindfold was placed over the patient's eyes as she was told that this may prevent a spinal headache, and then I switched places with the private attending doctor to sit in the doctor's delivery chair opposite the patient's vagina while the private doctor kept talking to the patient. I smiled at the young attending obstetrician and he smiled back at me. The delivery was smooth without the need for an episiotomy, a surgery to widen the vaginal space to avoid an irregular and uncontrolled tearing of the vagina as the baby's head stretched the vagina. The patient was relaxed in a twilight anesthesia state, with an anesthesiologist administering small doses of medication to reduce pain and create a mild amnesia of the birthing process and its pain.

Of course, now I realize that the powerful sedatives and anesthetics given to the woman in labor, even in small doses, also seeped into the placenta and all other bodily tissues and thus into the infant, interfering with breathing and other essential activities. This was why we had to get the infant delivered quickly and immediately cut the cord and transfer the baby to the waiting pediatrician for evaluation and to get an Apgar score, and then get the infant to the nursery where a trained staff of obstetrical nurses would oversee the newborn's condition.

If the infant was drowsy but breathing well this would affect its ability to nurse and be fed by the mother, another disruption of the natural course of childbirth and maternal bonding, in addition to missing the excellent nutrition and immune transfers from the first breast milk, called colostrum, loaded with important immune particles. Now we also know that the last blood from the umbilical cord has a large number of important stem cells that can help support the health of the baby, possibly even into adulthood.

After the Second World War, there was actually a movement to use baby formula instead of breast milk, at least for the people who could afford it. Sterile formula was considered more hygienic than having a baby put its mouth on the mother's skin, which was obviously not sterilized!

It seems that in medicine and most other fields as well, we humans tend to think we are smarter than Nature. But I did have a chance to see how childbirth should be done when I did home deliveries just as a midwife would do, without sedation and with a normal squatting birthing position.

I arrived with my wife at the home of one laboring woman and was greeted by her parents and taken into the living room where she was reclining comfortably with lots of pillows and towels. She smiled and we greeted each other. I had examined her several times as part of her prenatal evaluation, and she knew my wife, too. We had discussed hospital delivery vs. home delivery and possible risks, and she was totally dedicated to having her baby as naturally as possible.

Then I met her husband who was completely nude, sitting on the floor directly in front of her. This being the '60s era, although the calendar said '70s, "back to the earth," no shame, etcetera, I was not bothered by this. I spoke to my patient and she told me she was moving along nicely with regular contractions and that she had not yet "broken her water," that is, the amniotic sac had not yet released amniotic fluid, which usually led to a quick delivery.

I continued to talk to the patient and family while the husband was rocking slowly in front of his wife, when suddenly, without warning, a veritable tsunami of greenish water splashed all over the husband, who gave a loud gasp, and we all started laughing at what had just happened, including the husband's wife and then the husband as he was handed towels to wipe the greenish amniotic fluid from his body. And sure enough within ten minutes the pregnant woman was squatting and "pushing" and the baby's head appeared at the vaginal opening. A few grunts later by the laboring woman had the infant "crowning" at the vagina, and I supported the head and allowed a slow delivery of the head and then the rest of the body.

The newborn was immediately alert and breathing normally and moving and I helped the mom get her baby and bring him to her breast where he quickly searched and found a nipple and started sucking, all while still attached to an actively pumping umbilical cord. The cord didn't have to be stretched since "coincidentally" it was long enough for the distance from the mother's lower abdomen to her breast. Everyone was so happy. When the question of who would cut the cord came up, I explained we would cut it when it was no longer pulsating and had shriveled, which took a few more minutes, and I let the dried-off husband do that. There was no need to clamp the lifeless cord at that point since it was like old cellophane and the cutting was bloodless. There was no blood from the vagina either, and in a few more minutes the new mother said she had a cramp, and a small, bloodless placenta, the "afterbirth," was delivered effortlessly without a drop of blood from the vagina.

My work was done. I told them to call me the next day, and this happy, sucking newborn would get the highest Apgar score possible. The next day I heard from the new mom. She thanked me so much for helping her have the wonderful birth experience and the healthy baby, and she then laughed and brought up the funny explosion of amniotic fluid all over her husband and I laughed, too.

The next delivery I attended was a little more complicated. My wife and I arrived at the apartment where the couple lived and were greeted by the husband whom I had never met before. He said he was glad that I came because his wife was having some problems. I went into the living room with him and saw her propped up on the floor over a few towels. She quickly told me that she had been "pushing" for an hour and there had been no progress. I examined her and felt a normal pulse and heart and lungs and then palpated her abdomen using the Leopold maneuvers to find out if the fetus was positioned properly with the head downward and I also felt the fetus moving.

I asked her how often her contractions were coming, and she said she wasn't sure but she was pushing all the time and she hadn't felt any progress. I considered that something was blocking her cervix from dilating and told her I would do an internal exam. I put a sterile glove on and examined her and noted that the cervix was very edematous and spongy, probably from all of her straining against an undilated cervix.

She told me that her water "broke" about an hour ago and she had read that the baby should be coming out quickly after that happened. I explained that wasn't always the case and that all of her straining had caused swelling around her cervix and I felt that if we waited her normal labor would soon begin and the cervix would dilate. I got her and her husband to relax and asked her to tell me when she got a contraction.

Within fifteen minutes she had a contraction and then others came in a regular pattern and then some very strong contractions. I told her to try pushing with the next one and she said she felt the baby moving. As the strong contractions continued we started to see signs of her dilated vagina and the baby's head.

Within ten minutes the head crowned and I put gentle pressure on the head to prevent an uncontrolled "popping" of the head through the vagina, and allowed for a gentle advancement of the baby until he was fully delivered and unbloodied and breathing well with lots of movement. I gave the baby to his mom and told her to put him on her chest. This newborn quickly shook his head in search of a nipple and got one and started sucking greedily.

The parents were very happy now and relaxed and then a smaller contraction occurred and the small afterbirth (placenta) was delivered, also bloodlessly. The question of cutting the umbilical cord came up and I said we would do this when all the blood was transferred from the cord. Within a few more minutes we cut the shrunken cord with no need to clamp it first since its function was over and it was empty of blood and totally collapsed. Seeing an unsedated young mom with her unsedated, active newborn was wonderful. I told them to keep the baby warm and to call me in the morning, or sooner if needed. As I left I noted that there was not one drop of blood on the white towels she had been lying on.

My younger sister was also my obstetrical patient more than twenty years later. She and her husband were living in our house and she wanted natural childbirth. She had one child several years earlier when she was living in a California commune, the "Source family," and she did that with two other Source women who had experience with childbirth, so I knew she was capable of uncomplicated vaginal birth and I agreed. Her pregnancy was well advanced when she arrived at my house, and when she was near her due date, I examined her abdomen manually and felt the fetal head in the correct downward position. A couple of weeks later she told me that her water broke and she was starting to have contractions.

It was evening and I said we should all go to bed and rest because she would probably have the baby at night or in the morning. When I awoke early in the morning I went to see her and she told me her contractions didn't seem right. She removed her blanket and I immediately saw an abnormal abdominal shape and on palpation the fetus was lying crosswise, a transverse presentation, and there was no way that I was going to deliver her at home. She got dressed and we went to the local general hospital where I knew all the doctors and called the chief of obstetrics. He responded quickly and said the obvious: "Let's get her ready for a C-section." Later that morning she had her newborn son at her breast. My friend the obstetrician never charged her for the delivery and neither did the hospital charge her, and that was how old-fashioned professional courtesy worked in that era. My nephew is now a father and has a younger brother also by C-section, and both have an older sister born in the commune.

Chapter Fifteen - Private Practice

Finally, after all those years of training, working with other doctors, internship, two residencies, moonlighting, mini practices part time, I would have my own full-time specialty practice in a small growing city in Orange County, New York. I had never run a business but it seemed simple enough. Rent or buy a space, get the equipment and furniture you need, get malpractice insurance, hire a secretary, post a note in the local paper about your practice, meet the established doctors who would refer patients to you and then wait for the doorbell to ring. How could that be hard compared to doing surgery? And luckily it wasn't too hard. One glitch was the cost of the basic equipment I would need. I was broke at this time after an amicable divorce settlement with my first wife.

A friend recommended a local bank for a loan, and I met with the banker who wanted to know what my assets were and how much I needed. I explained that I didn't have much assets except a five-year-old car, but once I started practicing I should have no problem paying off a loan. He asked me how much I needed and I told him $5,000. He told me that I was asking for a large amount for someone just starting a medical practice. Then he asked me how much I thought I would earn in my first year and I told him what the senior doctors I questioned about this had said: $40,000 to $50,000. He laughed and said that he had been working at the bank for twenty years and didn't earn anything near that.

I explained that I was a board-eligible ENT doctor able to perform many different types of operations. I was trained at the prestigious New York Eye and Ear Infirmary in Manhattan where I was chief resident. We went back and forth for a while and he finally relented and gave me the loan and then said, a little too loudly, "Good luck," as I left the bank. I bought top-of-the-line equipment as my mentors had recommended, and they lasted through fifty years of practice. I never had to replace any of this basic and durable equipment.

My first secretary only lasted one month, but after that I had an excellent secretary who always did her best and was a great asset to my practice over the next decade. I also had my fiancée working in my office, and she was like a present-day physician assistant who was able to do many things that a doctor would do, such as ear washes for impacted ear wax, audiometry, surgical assisting and virtually anything else I taught her. Later in my career she also acted as a scrub nurse and was great at that job, too, and all of this without advanced training or certification, which shows what a dedicated intelligent person is capable of doing with the right motivation.

My practice quickly grew to a level that tested my endurance with an on-call schedule that included urgent surgeries at 2 A.M., plus weekend and holiday work.

My surgical schedule often involved three or four operations a day in addition to office hours and hospital meetings. My office assistant, now my wife, did get time off to have our two beautiful children. Luckily I survived! One long workday had us seeing and treating eighty-three patients, including post-ops, follow-ups and new patients, including biopsies and removal of nasal polyps and audiometry. Lunch was on the run, one bite of a sandwich and then back to work. That day was 7:30 A.M. to 10 P.M. and I was totally drained that night. We never booked anywhere near that many patients again for one day.

This was a very enervating practice, and after one decade I suffered burnout and ultimately sought a less controlling practice. I found a young doctor to take over the practice and I left with a few of my patients feeling abandoned but most of them wishing me good luck. And I did pay off that $5,000 loan in record time. My patients were very appreciative of my treatment. My exams and in-office treatments were as gentle as possible. I always pictured myself in the exam chair and how I would like to be treated.

Often a patient's spouse would be in the exam room during the exam and treatment and then the spouse would ask if he or she could have the same exam and treatment. This happened particularly when it came to earwax removal and the spouse saw how gentle I was, compared to times earwax removal with other doctors had been painful, or even bloody. I accommodated them since they were already in the office, and we would deal with the very simple paperwork at the end of the visit.

And then there were times when female patients would flirt with me and want to have a date with me or even something more immediate. In medical school we learned about the powerful effect of transference, where the doctor would become a love object instead of keeping the usual distance of the doctor-patient relationship. And remember, these encounters occurred during the '70s, which were not too far from the sexual revolution of the '60s and women's liberation, and birth control pills. Some of the young women had experienced quick "hookups" and why not with a young doctor? Not many patients were aware that my wife worked in the office. I would explain that I was married and that would usually end the flirtation.

One day the husband of a patient I had recently taken care of came to my office for an ear exam and told me that his wife wanted to have sex with me and he wouldn't mind since they already were swingers and switched couples on a regular basis. I declined the offer saying that his wife was really lovely but I was married. There was also one patient who flirted with me and thought I flirted, too, and the next time she came into the office for a post-op checkup she was dressed for a party with lots of makeup and expected to have a lunch date with me. When I seemed surprised that she thought we had agreed to the date, she got upset as if I were mocking her and tried to sue me for malpractice related to her recent successful operation. Her attorney sent me a request for medical records, and I had described her advances in my notes and there was never any lawsuit.

Malpractice lawsuits were a continuous hazard for doctors in the '70s. Previously malpractice occurred when the wrong leg was amputated or the surgeon operated while drunk resulting in a serious and unexpected complication. But it became common to get sued if the patient thought the operative result was not perfect. One other way for a doctor to get sued is if a cancer was not diagnosed immediately after a patient left the office and failed to return for a recommended test and reexamination in a month, and then a year later that patient sees another doctor who makes a diagnosis of cancer. Many of these lawsuits were what the older doctors called "nuisance" or "frivolous" lawsuits. I was sued three times for persistent pain after nasal surgery when I asked for payment of a bill, and then when it wasn't paid I sent the bill to collection. The suit was always dropped when I canceled the unpaid debt.

Interestingly, the attorney's subpoenas always started with "Ronald Halweil, MD, willfully and maliciously injured" etcetera. Some aggressive doctors would even countersue the patient over these nuisance lawsuits. Malpractice insurance premiums continued to rise in the '70s. For a while they doubled every two years, starting at $2,000 per year, then $4,000, then $8,000, then $16,000, all the way to $40,000, and the doctors raised their fees accordingly and had marches on Albany to get the governor involved. This was especially burdensome for obstetricians who paid double what surgeons paid for insurance, and many of them gave up delivering babies entirely since all birth defects were considered to be due to delivery complications or prenatal errors by the ob-gyn doctor. Many of these doctors gave up obstetrics and just focused their practices on gynecology, and that also drastically reduced their malpractice insurance premiums.

The problems with liability insurance and malpractice suits persist today, and the concept of "tort reform" has never been fully realized as a way to reduce frivolous malpractice cases. This would be an easy way to reduce medical insurance costs and would probably lower the cost of medical care in general. Of course people truly injured by doctors' treatments or the treatments of other health care providers would get all care and treatment for recovery. Medical professionals would be involved in assessing the injuries and could interview any health care provider to assess the reasons for the problem and if necessary make changes to the provider's privileges. Of course any doctor who "willfully and maliciously" injured a patient should go to jail!

One of the best head and neck cancer surgeons during this era, the one who took cases that no one else would touch because they were too complex, and they lacked his experience and operative skills, was the recipient of many lawsuits but was inevitably declared innocent in court. Even today there are hospitals and doctors that avoid complicated cases in order to show better survival and cure scores for their surgeries and get higher local and national rankings.

It took months for me to find a new practice. I saw doctors who were retiring and asking what I thought were very high prices to take over their practices, and others were out of state, which seemed very inconvenient for my wife and growing children. Finally, a doctor who had been in ENT residency with me suggested a small city in New Jersey where he was raised, not far from where we were living in Manhattan, and after checking it out and walking through the neighborhoods, I was reminded of Brooklyn when I was growing up. They even had outdoor fruit markets, nice tree-lined streets that were clean and a medium-size general hospital where I could operate on my patients as needed.

I met with senior doctors in the hospital and learned that although there were several ENT doctors, none had the prestigious set of credentials I had, nor the letters of recommendation from internationally respected ear, nose and throat doctors, such as Dr. Samuel Rosen, who developed the stapes operation for otosclerosis deafness, and pioneering plastic surgeons that I had worked with at the New York Eye and Ear Infirmary. At this point in my career I was a "seasoned" doctor who had done well over 1,000 operations. Basically I was in the "sweet spot" for a surgeon. I had excellent vision, steady hands and the strength to operate for hours, and I was only in my early forties.

I met with the chief of surgery, and he was impressed with all the endorsements from doctors I had worked with in the past. Everyone seemed happy with me except for the other ear, nose and throat doctors in the community since I represented competition, but I would become friendly with all of them over time. My first office was small, and luckily I quickly met and hired a secretary who had worked at another medical office in town. She was smart and efficient and the practice grew rapidly on word of mouth and referrals from other doctors. But I did need more space, and there was a house with an office attached that had just become available after the death of the doctor living and practicing there. The house was large and the office was spacious and separated from the house by one large door. I looked at the house and office and realized that this would be ideal with plenty of room if my family chose to leave Manhattan where we were living. I bought the house and I became the fourth doctor to practice in that house since the early 1900s when it was built by the first certified general surgeon in that city.

The hospital was a fifteen-minute walk from the house, so I didn't even have to drive a car there. From Manhattan I did the reverse commute, so I was able to start office hours as early as 7:00 or 7:30 and I would see the first two patients before my secretary came to the office. For some patients that early morning appointment was a necessary convenience for them so they could get to work on time. I had a good kitchen in the house and I would prepare my lunch and take a one-hour lunch break, something I was never able to do in my first private practice. Patients were spaced at reasonable intervals and new patients would get up to half an hour or even more to give their medical history, followed by the examination and the consultation afterward, when I would make a diagnosis and recommend treatments. I was always interested in patients who had seen several other doctors before me without a good diagnosis, including seeing "top doctors."

I found that when a patient is not rushed, the history taking is more productive, and the face-to-face time made this less stressful for the patient and more honest. Often something the patient would say reminded me of a case I had seen or heard of and I could ask more pertinent questions and arrive at the aha! moment where the patient says, "That's right," and we'd both smile and I'd recommend effective treatment and a follow-up appointment. Cases like that always made me feel like Sherlock Holmes solving a difficult crime.

Compare that with our modern history, talking with the doctor on the computer documenting the history, answering all the standard mandated questions in the electronic medical record format and only occasionally seeing the patient face to face, with limited time to perform the physical exam, make a diagnosis and then recommend treatment. My consultation room was spacious and airy with three large windows and the possibility of fresh air on all mild weather days.

I adopted the custom of giving patients most of the common medications they would need after my diagnosis at no charge since these were well-known medications, such as Sudafed, steroid creams, amoxicillin, antibiotic ear drops and allergy pills. I was able to buy them in quantity for a small fraction of their retail cost. This saved time and money for the patient, and they were able to start treatments immediately. I learned about this when I worked with a famous Viennese ENT doctor with a thriving private practice in New York City.

My surgical practice at the new hospital was very convenient, too. I always wanted an early start since I then had better control of the whole day, which also included my office practice. I would walk to the hospital and after greeting the nurses and other doctors I would head to my locker to change into surgical scrubs. I always arrived early but sometimes there would be a delay when one of the members of the operating team was late or the patient wasn't moved from the hospital bed on time, but usually this delay was under fifteen minutes.

Once everyone was in the operating room we could start. If the operation was under local anesthesia it was easier for me. But at least half of the operations at that time in the mid-1980s were under general or fractional anesthesia, which meant another important doctor was in the operating room, the anesthesiologist. I had worked with anesthesiologists and nurse anesthetists for years, and if I was lucky enough to work with very good ones, I would ask for them for future cases, since they knew my techniques, and I knew their skill. In a similar manner the surgical assistant who stood opposite me at the operating table was an important part of surgery and I was always happier to have the assistant I knew and who knew my techniques as well.

As surgeon I was the "captain" of the team and responsible for every part of the operation, and there were times when it seemed that these other people in the operating room were sabotaging me. Once I was doing a nasal and sinus operation on a young man and everything was going well. The patient had asked for general anesthesia by saying that he wanted to be "put out" for the surgery that I could have done easily under local anesthesia. The surgery went well and finally all suturing and packing was in place and we waited for the patient to come out of anesthesia and be moved to a gurney and transported to the recovery room so my next patient could be prepared for surgery.

After five minutes there was no sign that the patient was waking up, which was nerve wracking because occasionally a patient would have a genetic predisposition that made them unable to detoxify the anesthesia and that patient would be anesthetized for a long time. After twenty minutes I happened to look at the anesthesiologist's table and noticed that the patient was still receiving nitrous oxide! So although the primary anesthetic was off, my patient was still asleep with this other common anesthetic. I quickly told the anesthesiologist and he said, "Oops," and stopped the nitrous.

Obviously I was very upset but also very relieved that there was a simple solution to the problem. Within minutes the patient was awake and we transferred him to the recovery room. At another time this same anesthesiologist was working with me on a cosmetic nasal surgery on a young woman. In the past I did these operations under local anesthesia, but at this time most patients opted for general anesthesia, and that was what she got.

The operation went smoothly and I had finished most of it when all of a sudden blood started gushing out of her nose from every spot I had worked on, something I had never seen before in a thousand operations. My careful surgeries usually had minimal bleeding since I used local anesthetic as well as the general anesthetic and that reduced bleeding. I applied pressure to all the areas of the nose, but it did not reduce the bleeding. I was ready to call for blood to transfuse the patient and I called out to the anesthesiologist and asked what was happening. He quickly moved and I could see him changing some dials on his anesthesia equipment that had caused a rapid rise in her blood pressure with consequent hemorrhage. The bleeding slowed and then stopped and I was able to finish the operation without transfusing any blood.

Once again from being frightened and horrified, I was happy that this patient survived the operation and never needed a transfusion. Since this was the same anesthesiologist who had kept my patient anesthetized for a long time after an operation was over by carelessly allowing continued nitrous oxide anesthesia, I told the chief of anesthesia that I didn't want to work with this doctor anymore, and he understood.

Another anesthesiologist at another time was not paying attention to my patient getting cosmetic eyelid surgery who did not want local anesthesia, which would have been the best way to do this operation. The operation went very well and I finished the delicate suturing of the eyelid incisions when the patient suddenly started choking on the endotracheal tube as the anesthesia wore off. The anesthesiologist was supposed to quickly remove the tube at that point, but he wasn't at the head of the operating table. The patient continued to strain against her endotracheal tube as her eyes bulged and started bleeding and then I saw him running to the patient and giving her more anesthesia to relax her struggling and stop her choking. At that point my greatest fear was that all that choking and bleeding might compromise her vision, that she might have bled into her eyes, and I quickly removed those carefully applied sutures and palpated her eyes to feel if there was increased pressure and they felt normal to me. The bleeding from the incisions stopped and I cleaned her lids and cheeks and started resuturing the eyelid incisions. The anesthesiologist apologized for not being at the head of the table to quickly extubate the patient as she was gaining consciousness.

As I was suturing, I noticed that blood had even gotten under the cheek skin closest to the lower lids and that meant lots of post-op bruising, and I had assured her that there would be very little bruising with my careful technique. I followed her back as they wheeled her to the recovery room since I was still worried most about loss of vision and even blindness and I pictured the end of my surgical career, too.

I waited in the recovery room for her to wake up so I could determine if her vision had changed, and happily she saw me clearly but asked why I was there. At her post-op visits she wondered why there was so much bruising since I had assured her that there would be very little bruising. Later, when the bruising was gone she told me how happy she was with her youthful eyelids.

And then there was the case of a young blond girl with creamy white skin on the operating table for a tonsillectomy. The anesthesiologist had anesthetized her enough with an anesthesia mask to insert the endotracheal tube. I turned away for a second to ask for a special instrument, and when I looked back her face was purple. I immediately knew that he had put the tube in her esophagus instead of her trachea and she was not getting any oxygen. I immediately alerted the anesthesiologist and he quickly removed the tube and reinserted it properly and her face instantaneously lost its purple color and became pure white again. This was a very serious error, a life and death error, and I was shaken up about it.

I spoke to the chief of surgery and told him what happened and he explained that the anesthesiologist was taking new medication for high blood pressure and anyway he was retiring in three months. I told him I didn't want him on any more of my cases and he said okay. And then there was the time the anesthesiologist and the nurse dropped the young girl I had just operated on for enlarged adenoids. They dropped her as they were transferring her from the operating table to the gurney to get her to the recovery room.

She bruised her cheek and was getting a black eye when they told me, with apologies, that she had somehow wiggled out of their grip.

We got facial x-rays and saw no fractures, but then I had to explain to the parents why she had this injury, not an easy job. I emphasized that there was no fracture, and the bruising wouldn't last more than a few days. The operating room nurse supervisor actually blamed me for the accident because I was not there to help them transfer her to the gurney. Whatever happens in the operating room has always been the responsibility of the surgeon!

Thankfully these anesthesia problems were not common and I worked with excellent doctors and nurse anesthetists who were able to detect problems before they became serious, especially with a condition called "malignant hyperthermia." This genetic condition can be triggered by anesthesia and is more common in children. If the anesthesiologist is paying attention, they can recognize it by increased heart rate and quickly give an antidote, but you can tell by the name "malignant" that there was a time when it was not commonly known and surgeons would explain the death of a child by saying the child couldn't tolerate the anesthesia. Twice in my career anesthesiologists recognized the earliest symptoms of this awful condition and immediately gave the antidote and saved the day.

Many of my referrals for surgery came from the operating room nurses and from the emergency room and recovery room nurses who saw firsthand my skills as an operator and how comfortable my patients were as they recovered from surgery compared to the patients of other doctors.

One emergency room nurse was amazed that the children I treated for facial lacerations never cried. And I explained to her that I spent time talking to the children and told them I would not hurt them, and I would drip a few drops of local anesthetic into the wound and wait a couple of minutes before I injected a small amount of the anesthetic into the wound from the raw inside where I had dropped some of the local. I kept talking to the child who was now more relaxed because there was no pain. I continued this slow advancement of the local anesthetic until the entire wound was anesthetized, at which point I cleaned the wound with hydrogen peroxide and sterile gauze pads, carefully, then sutured the wound and applied a dressing and told the child they were very good and I would see them at my office in a few days. The parents who had been waiting outside the ER room were amazed that there was no crying and thanked me. I told them to call my office to get the appointment for suture removal and wound evaluation in a few days.

At this time in my practice I needed a new secretary since my original secretary had to leave for family reasons. Once again I quickly hired a bright and conscientious secretary who was a great asset in my office and stayed with me until the end of this private practice.

House calls by a doctor were already a thing of the past, except for very special patients when I started doing them. My office patients would tell me about "shut-ins" they knew who couldn't hear and asked if they could be brought to my office by ambulance for treatment. That idea seemed a little extravagant and wasteful to me and I suggested a house call, something I used to get from my pediatrician who was also our family doctor in that era. I was always impressed with this doctor who would come to our apartment in any weather if I or my mom was too sick to go to his office, and now I had the opportunity to do a house call as a specialist.

If the address was less than ten blocks from my office, I would pack my black leather doctor's bag that I got in medical school and head off walking to the patient's home. If they were further away I would drive to the house. The patient's family would greet me at the door and then I would be brought to the bedridden person. I was impressed with how well these disabled people were cared for.

One woman who had been bedridden with paralysis for thirty years never had one bedsore, a tribute to the care the relatives gave her. I examined the ears with my portable otoscope and saw both ears clogged with dry ear wax, basically a complete seal of both ear canals. I removed some of the wax with a stainless-steel curette and then asked the women to get me a bowl of warm water so I could irrigate the canals to remove the wax with a classic German-made ear syringe I used for my whole career.

The patient couldn't sit up, so I kneeled on a folded towel and had one of the women hold a plastic ear cup made for this procedure under the ear to catch the runoff as I squirted warm water into the canal and watched the debris flow into the cup, then I used my otoscope to see if the canal was clear. If I saw that it was not clear, I needed to repeat this again to get the rest of the wax out to enable me to see the eardrum. I did the same procedure on the opposite ear and saw the patient smile when her sisters spoke near her ears: She could hear now! They thanked me and I left with the billing information for Medicare.

I continued to do house calls every other week with two to three hours set aside for this, and then returned to my office to see patients until closing time. I got personal satisfaction from this activity even though I lost income by not seeing patients in my office. Medicare allowed a double payment for house calls but discontinued that extra fee two years after I started this service.

I felt a strong connection to this community I worked in.

I treated the police, the firefighters, nurses, doctors and dentists and clergy. The insurance companies paid well for my work, and I supported local institutions like the library. One year I paid for new bulletproof vests for the police, anonymously. I saw my patients when I walked on the streets or shopped in the stores. When I wrote a book on food and health, the local newspaper wrote about it and many of my patients and their friends bought my book. This was all to change with the advent of the HMO (health maintenance organization).

I was working in the time before the HMO corporations took over traditional private practice with reduced fees for the doctors, which resulted in constraints in the doctor's time to spend with patients and a common four patients per hour schedule. When the HMO was in its infancy and most doctors didn't fully understand its function, the doctors at the hospital I was affiliated with were invited to an educational program on the HMO benefits for the physician and we were told that refreshments would be provided. This meeting was held at a conference room in our hospital that could accommodate at least thirty doctors.

We were all interested to find out about the innovative system of getting patients referred by a corporation although we had heard that the payments were low. The moderator was a well-dressed spokesperson for the new Prudential HMO company and he extolled the benefits of having a steady stream of patients and a guaranteed prompt payment. Most of the doctors in attendance already had a steady stream of patients who usually paid their bills promptly at the time of the visit, so we wanted to find out why this new paradigm would benefit us. The HMO representative passed around informational sheets with the most common visit fees and the fees of the most common procedures and operations we would be doing.

The room got quiet as we carefully checked all the "codes" that applied to our practices, and then a murmur started as we talked with those doctors sitting near us, people we already knew from working at the hospital. The murmur grew, and finally someone called out that these fees were very low compared to what we already charged, so why would we want to join this company? The moderator calmly said that we would benefit by having more patients, and then someone called out that we already had enough patients and then there was some laughter. At this point the previously smiling speaker had a grim face and pointed a shaking finger at us saying, "In a few years, you'll wish you got even half of these generous fees." He got off the stage and left while we were stunned at this unexpected nasty turn-around and just a little frightened by his prediction of our future.

Within a few years we started to feel the power of HMOs as they took over the way doctors practiced medicine, and we sure would have enjoyed those original fees the spokesman had shown us at that hospital meeting. A group of us decided that we should meet for discussions about the future of our practices and the future of medicine in general and that we should find ways to save money on office supplies by purchasing in bulk. We also told each other stories we heard about HMOs, some of them quite humorous while others were distressing. We had all been friends for years and we spoke about family, kids growing up, and also about how we were saving for retirement.

Then to make matters much worse, the U.S. Department of Justice contacted the busiest doctors in the community, which included me and the other doctors who made up our little monthly meetings, and issued a fine of $1 million for the crime of "restraint of trade." The HMOs had noted that the busiest doctors in our community were not signing up with the HMOs at the same rate as surrounding communities were and suspected that we were "conspiring" to avoid joining the HMOs. We were interviewed by government agents, and we denied the charges, but we were still liable for the fine. We were told that the fine would be dropped if we signed up with the HMOs, or we could hire attorneys and fight the federal government's judgment. Of course we signed up.

Luckily for us, there were still a large number of patients who were not in HMOs, but that amount continued to dwindle. For me in my specialty practice, patients in HMO plans were not able to see specialists without a referral from their primary care doctor, and this eliminated many of my patients. The surgical part of my practice was discontinued after I did the math and discovered that the malpractice cost of doing an operation was greater than the HMO or Medicare payments for most of the operations I performed.

Ultimately I closed my no longer "private" practice and joined a nice group of internists and family doctors whom I knew. That worked well for a long time until a possible embezzlement bankrupted the group and it was taken over by a doctor no one knew. At least for me, working conditions became very unpleasant as he reduced the share of payments for my work that I had signed up for by saying he was losing too much money every month and he had no other option.

As I left this wonderful group of young doctors who had become my friends and colleagues and they had a farewell party for me, I entered the last phase of my medical career.

Chapter Sixteen - My Heart Disease

My family, on both sides, has a terrible history of heart disease. Our intensive education in the new field of genetics during medical school made it seem that at conception, our destiny has been set in stone. My dad's father died at forty of a heart attack, my mom's dad died in his fifties after several heart attacks. My dad developed heart disease in his early fifties and had a coronary artery bypass operation in his mid-fifties. The coronary artery bypass was so new at that time that no thoracic surgeon in New York City had more than a single-digit experience with the surgery.

I sent my dad to a great cardiac surgeon in Texas, Dr. Denton Cooley. He had lectured us in medical school on the new field of cardiovascular surgery and he answered my phone call and told me, in that great Texas accent, "Send your dad down here Dr. Halweil and we'll fix him up and send him back to you in a week." And he sure did. He told my dad the importance of exercising, something he was never interested in, and after nearly six pleasant post-op years, he became symptomatic again and had frequent visits to the emergency room before he succumbed to his heart disease and died at sixty-two. His younger brother had two coronary artery bypasses and survived to seventy-two. I thought I would have an early death, too, although there were some indications that coronary artery disease could be reversed with a low-fat diet, exercise and weight loss if needed.

Nathan Pritikin, although not a doctor, researched and wrote about the origins of this common heart disease and how it could be reversed, and Dr. Dean Ornish was also writing about this, as well as the interestingly named Dr. Dock who wrote about this, too.

I was in my mid-forties, with a wife and two growing children and a busy medical/surgical practice, when I had the first inkling of heart disease with irregular heartbeats that occurred when I would lie down to go to sleep. If I sat up they would go away, but as soon as I would lie down again they would return.

After a week of this, I went to see a cardiologist I was friendly with at the hospital where I worked. He asked me if I had chest pain or shortness of breath, which I did not have, and I told him my family history, which was full of heart disease. His exam was thorough and he ordered lab tests, especially cholesterol and other lipids. He tried to give me an in-office stress test, but it quickly showed a cardiographic irregularity and he stopped it even though I had no chest pain or shortness of breath.

I went for my blood tests but also started to think that my lifestyle had changed over the last dozen years, with weight gain and lack of regular exercise. I practiced near a wonderful old-fashioned Italian bakery, and was a daily customer for their delicious cookies and other pastries, a real deviation from the lifestyle I had for many years. I made up my mind to live a healthier life, following the guidelines of Pritikin, Ornish and Dr. Dock.

After looking at the blood tests, my cardiologist said I had a very high cholesterol of 300 with mostly LDL, which was considered "bad" cholesterol, as well as very high lipids. He made an appointment for me to have the best noninvasive heart test available, the thallium stress test, and told me I was not to exercise at all since my lab tests and failed office stress test showed I could be in danger of sudden cardiac death, but I was allowed to walk short distances. And he emphasized no eating on the morning of the test, which was three days off.

I was enjoying my new dietary regimen, mostly vegetables, fruits and whole grains, and I was being more active, taking longer walks at a good speed, and I wanted to do more. I didn't like the prohibition of exercise and couldn't conceive of being on a treadmill without practicing, so I went to the gym where I still had a membership and got on a treadmill at a medium speed for ten minutes and it felt good, although I had a fear that my doctor's warning of sudden cardiac death could happen. I had no chest pain or shortness of breath, but I ended the "workout" for the day.

The next day I was on the treadmill at medium speed again but for a longer time and even got sweaty but felt good throughout the workout. I was still enjoying my new diet, and my wife was helping me stay on the tastiest low-fat vegetable diet. The day before the thallium treadmill test, I did a more vigorous treadmill test for myself and once again felt good with the exercise without any discomfort.

When I got to the lab the next day for the stress test I was greeted by my cardiologist and set up for the testing event with electrodes attached to my chest to continually monitor my heart. The treadmill started slowly but gradually increased in speed, all the while my doctor asking if I had any chest pain while he told me that the cardiogram was showing signs of cardiac ischemia (the heart muscle not getting enough oxygen-carrying blood). Then the treadmill changed from flat and went up to incline and the speed of the treadmill increased, all the while I was asked if I had any chest pain. This gradual speeding and rising incline continued until the doctor said we were nearing the end of the test and I could stop if I wanted, but I said I would like to continue, although at this point I felt like I was running uphill. And then it was over and I was breathing heavily and sweating.

My doctor said he was surprised that I was able to finish the treadmill. The thallium was injected and the nurse took off the electrodes. I was told that I had a free period and could go home and the doctor would call me with the results in a few hours.

I was happy to go home and shower and eat while I waited for the test results.

When I got the expected call, my doctor sounded frantic and told me the scan showed that I had no blood flow in my left anterior descending artery, the main blood supply to the heart muscle itself, also called the "widow-maker," and that I could die at any time now and must come to the hospital immediately for treatment. I told him I felt fine and if my heart was not getting any blood how come I'm standing here and talking to you on the phone. He said that doesn't matter and I have to drop everything and take a cab to the hospital and he will be waiting with his team to do a coronary angiogram and balloon angioplasty of the totally blocked artery. I said I would like to wait until my wife and kids come home in an hour to talk to them about this procedure. Once again he said that I had no time for that, I'm a walking "time bomb" and I must get to the hospital as soon as possible.

At this point our conversation became very repetitive as he kept emphasizing the urgency of this situation and the possibility of sudden death. I kept saying I felt fine and I want to wait at least until I talk to my wife and that we can talk more soon and I had to go now. I thanked him and said I'm hanging up for now. When my wife got home and I told her the story she was frightened but also asked how I could look so good and feel fine if this was such an emergency.

There was data coming out at this time that the coronary balloon angioplasty only worked for a matter of months and then needed to be repeated or a major coronary artery bypass procedure could be done. This was before cardiac stents. I reassured my wife and kids that I felt great and I performed the full stress test without any discomfort even though it was quite strenuous. We decided that I didn't have to rush into this and we should get a second opinion, and I would continue on my Pritikin diet, exercise and weight loss while I sought other cardiologist opinions.

I got recommendations for several New York City cardiologists and made an appointment to see one, which was rather brief because after the history and the exam he said that he would only take me as a patient if I had a coronary angiogram first, and he had to do that or else he would be liable for malpractice by not following community standards. As a practicing physician, I understood what he said and I respected his position and thanked him as I left the office. The next doctor I saw was a repeat of the former. He could not have me as a patient unless I had an angiogram first.

I was getting frustrated at this point, although I was feeling stronger and healthier with each passing day with my exercise regimen and new diet. I saw the last doctor on the list, and he understood what I was doing and commended me for my lifestyle change. He did a thorough exam and also gave me an in-office stress test where he noted the same electrocardiographic abnormality but saw that my breathing was good and I had no chest pain. He would take me as a patient and he prescribed a statin medication, a low-dose beta blocker and a low-dose aspirin regimen, and he would see me again after a new round of lab tests. This doctor was also a runner and had changed his lifestyle when he developed cardiac symptoms years before.

I had regular visits with this doctor, which always included a stress test, but I had my lab tests for cholesterol nearer to my office. Although my overall cholesterol levels were much reduced, the ratio of HDL to LDL never changed and every doctor I spoke with about this said it was genetic and I had to live with this as I maintained my healthy lifestyle. After taking the statin medication for a few years, I finally had to stop due to the severe leg cramps, and I also stopped getting regular blood tests as well since they never changed and anyway my total cholesterol was much lower than the 300 I originally had.

I was feeling healthier than I had for years, my running speed had improved and my running schedule was carefully followed with very few exceptions. I had gotten down to a weight I hadn't seen in years and everyone associated me with "being healthy" and wished they could be as conscientious about health as I was. The original arrhythmias that were the start of this healthy program were gone and I stopped going to my cardiologist on a regular basis.

I enjoyed my medical practice and my family and my fishing hobby, which put lots of fresh fish on the family table, and I gave fish to neighbors and friends, too. One morning I had to get blood tests for an updated life insurance policy. The nurse who took care of this also commented on my normal blood pressure and regular heart rhythm and weight and asked me if I was a runner and I smiled and said yes.

I asked her if I could get a copy of the lab tests, and she said it would be mailed to me. When I got the test results I was astonished to see that my HDL to LDL ratio had totally reversed itself, so instead of an HDL in the 20s, it was now in the 70s, and the LDL was in the

40s, a real shock to me as a doctor, since I had been told by every cardiologist that this was impossible. This certainly reinforced the concept that the body could heal itself if proper diet, exercise and general lifestyle were adopted. My wife always felt it also had to do with the piece of very dark chocolate and half glass of red wine that she insisted I have daily.

My fifties and sixties were a time of amazing vigor and health for me. I was still running two or three times a week on a beach close to our weekend house in Southampton, even in the dead of winter. I was surf fishing from March to December and seldom returned home without fish, which became an integral part of my diet. Gardening was now on my list, especially growing raspberries and blackberries as well as herbs and mustard. Other crops invariably were eaten by deer or smaller animals. I commuted to work at my New Jersey office, and then later on to my teaching position at the New York Eye and Ear Infirmary in Manhattan, my alma mater.

I had a new cardiologist at this time at Mount Sinai. I was occasionally bothered by arrhythmia again and I thought it wise to get an evaluation. This internationally known cardiologist in charge of the cardiac department took my history and examined me and ordered blood tests, and when I returned to see him he recommended the latest radioactive isotope stress test, which I completed without shortness of breath or chest pains, and although the cardiogram while I was on the treadmill showed the usual irregularities, the radioactive isotope study showed good blood flow to my heart possibly related to collateral arteries, which added extra oxygen-rich blood to my heart. These smaller arteries were likely a result of my exercise regimen stimulating their growth and development.

My doctor recommended that I stop taking the small dose of beta blocker, which I had been on for years, saying that my heart rate was already low due to my regular exercise, and the medication may be adding to the slowing of the heart rate and causing the arrhythmia. He told me to enjoy my life and return as needed.

When I had my seventieth birthday, there was a big fuss with celebration, even my sister who lived in Washington State made the trip to congratulate me, quite a pleasant surprise to me. Round numbers ending in zero are always given more attention on birthdays with somewhat less excitement at the half numbers in between the zeros. My early seventies didn't feel much different than my sixties, but there were changes. Afternoon naps became more important, and I felt the loss of the nap when I worked through the afternoon into early evening during my teaching stint at the New York Eye and Ear twice a week.

I loved helping the young doctors, but I didn't enjoy all of the typing involved in electronic medical records, which was very fatiguing for me. I found myself thinking more and more about retirement. I joked about my "bucket list," which had only one wish, to retire before I died, which some people thought was humorous while others thought it was macabre.

One chilly and rainy late winter's evening, I left the hospital carrying a small bag of organic foods I had bought at lunchtime to take to our apartment. The streets were crowded with people rushing to the subway stations in the dark and I was moving quickly to get out of the rain, when I felt a tightness in my chilled body, especially my left chest and arm, which I thought might be angina. I slowed down and that relieved some of the discomfort. I really wanted shelter at the subway station, still two blocks away, but as soon as I picked up the pace, the chest and arm discomfort returned. I walked slowly to the subway entrance and felt better when I got out of the cold and the rain.

I felt normal when I got to the apartment and had dinner with my wife but thought it might be time to see my cardiologist again, and I saw him the following week. He was happy to see me but asked why I hadn't been back in nine years. I reminded him that after the last visit he had told me to go enjoy my life and never gave me an appointment.

I told him the story of the chest pain on the cold and rainy night after an exhausting day, and he agreed with my diagnosis of angina. But when he examined me he found normal pulse and blood pressure and heart and lung sounds and normal cardiogram. I had done some research on something called cold weather angina, which I remembered learning about in medical school and told him about it. He said that with my family and personal history it might be wise to do an angiogram with stenting if obstruction was found. I asked if there was a noninvasive test I could get, and he suggested a coronary artery calcium CT scan and I agreed to this.

After the scan was performed, I asked to see the results with the radiologist. As a doctor I was permitted to do this rather than waiting several days for a result. The young doctor (actually most doctors seem young to me now) went over the calcium score and told me it was high. Up to 300 was considered normal and mine was very high at 3,000, and that surely got my attention. When my cardiologist got the results, he said that I should have the angiogram with possible stents and it could be done the following week. I told him that I was feeling fine and would like some time to consider this, and he said that would be all right but I should take a low-dose aspirin every other day.

I didn't return to his office for about nine months and told him I had no symptoms and was doing all my regular exercises without chest discomfort or shortness of breath. He said that new cardiac studies showed no difference in morbidity or mortality in people with asymptomatic heart disease with medical management or with stents and that he would like to see me in a year or sooner as needed. What a coincidence that the impressive ISCHEMIA heart study ("ischemia" means decreased blood flow anywhere in the body), was published at this time in my life. This advice was being followed by cardiologists including my cardiologist.

Chapter Seventeen - Eating Epidemic

It's hard to believe that eating, something we must do to stay alive, can be called an epidemic and a plague, but it has happened. Throughout human history food scarcity has generally been the big problem for people, with malnutrition, hunger and starvation and death.

How did this get reversed?
The hunter-gatherer phase of human history was dependent on the ready availability of sufficient edible plants and animals on a regular basis. This was the work of every man and woman in addition to finding shelter and water and avoiding becoming food for local carnivores. When local supplies of plant food and game were exhausted, migration was needed to satisfy thirst and hunger or else disaster would follow. Fast forward thousands of years, and we have advanced civilizations and agriculture as well as animal husbandry producing copious amounts of dietary needs so that starvation has become less of a problem except for some developing and war-torn countries.

As a result of these modern achievements, most people can eat as much as they want, or can afford, and starvation is no longer the great fear it used to be. One of the Four Horsemen of the Apocalypse has been controlled. Only pestilence, war and death itself are left.

So how did food become an epidemic?
Overeating has been an issue for as long as extra food has been available. People with great wealth and power were always able to buy as much food and drink as they wanted. Feasting was a pastime of the rich and powerful throughout the ages, and there was the gastric dis-

tress to deal with, which used to be called "dyspepsia," then called "heartburn," and now known as "GERD," gastroesophageal reflux disease.

For the average person, a celebration could trigger overeating and gastric distress, this tended to be the exception since large amounts of food would be very expensive. But the well-to-do and the powerful could afford this feasting on a regular basis and they would gain weight and develop chronic symptoms: indigestion, chest pains, shortness of breath, vision changes and so on.

Even thousands of years ago doctors recognized problems in these habitual overeaters. They needed to urinate frequently, needed to drink large amounts of water and continue to consume large amounts of food. They developed cramps, fatigue, weakness and many other symptoms. Their doctors tested their urine by taste and noted sweet urine, and because there were large amounts of this sweet urine, they named the disease diabetes mellitus, which translates to "large amounts of sweet urine," and we still use that name for the end result of the plague of overeating today.

The ancient Egyptian doctors were the first to record the disease they called "diabete," which translated to "syphon," since the amount of urine excreted was similar to liquid flowing from a syphon. The doctors also noted that wherever these patients urinated, ants and flies would be attracted to the urine. The Greeks, and through them the Romans, knew about this diabetes, too.

I was fortunate to have a private medical/surgical practice as an otolaryngologist in a small city for more than three consecutive decades. This gave me an opportunity that few doctors have had. I was able to see a child of ten, and then see him or her again at twenty and then again at thirty or forty. This continuity allowed me to observe something I didn't expect to see, and that was the change in body size over the years. It started very subtly but then my young patients returned to my office larger, overweight, taking various medications from their primary care physician and complaining to me about heartburn and snoring.

When I practiced medicine and surgery in the '70s, heartburn was something that people knew they were responsible for, caused by dysfunctional overeating or eating the wrong foods. They knew that they were to blame for the symptoms and only needed the willpower to improve their eating to avoid the distress. There were numerous remedies for heartburn, and they were advertised widely, for example Alka-Seltzer, Tums, Rolaids, Pepto-Bismol and sodium bicarbonate, to name a few common ones. And snoring was well known to be the "fat" man's problem, which could be ameliorated by weight loss. It was usually the wife who complained about snoring and another solution was to sleep in a separate bed from the snorer.

I often think back to the middle-age internist who lectured to us on diet in medical school. He told us that by the time anyone reaches adulthood they should know which foods agreed with them, and which did not, and all they needed to do was avoid those foods, or the quantity of other foods, in order to control their digestive symptoms.

Contrast this doctor's wisdom with the birth of the powerful "antacids" that were being promoted on TV with slick videos and commentary, such as, "Why aren't you eating this delicious pizza and spaghetti with spicy sauce? All you have to do is take this pill and you can enjoy all of this food you used to love," and this was with one sad man who wasn't eating at a table with many "roundish" people laughing and enjoying these tasty foods.

It wasn't only the heartburn or GERD or snoring that was the really dangerous problem. Many of my former normal-size patients were taking oral medications to control blood sugar and incipient type 2 diabetes. In medical school in the '60s we studied diabetes, but it was type 1 diabetes and it wasn't called type "1" because this second type of diabetes was not yet a fully recognized common disease. It was often called "adult onset diabetes," and even that had to be changed when children were being afflicted with it, so diabetes became type 1 and type 2.

Type 1 diabetes is a terrible disease that has a major hereditary component and caused the early death of many young people before the breakthrough of insulin production that was then used by injection to regulate blood sugar and allow the patient to lead a normal life.

Summertime was when I was able to most easily see the transformation of my once normal-size patients, since they came into the office with short-sleeve shirts or dresses that bared arms and legs, and I saw arms that were larger than the ones I used to see in the weightlifting gym I belonged to in the early '60s. And I also saw men who had the abdominal shape of pregnant women and I would quickly guess the month of gestation as I did when studying obstetrics in med school. I called this "male pregnancy," but it was really no laughing matter.

So in the relatively short space of thirty to forty years, there were much larger people on the streets and in my office, and the medical industry was starting to pay attention to this, especially the endocrinologists who were getting busier and busier evaluating and treating the pancreatic hormone disease called type 2 diabetes.

The industrial revolution changed how people lived, how they worked, moved and ate. No longer did people live the biblical prophecy of earning their bread by the sweat of their brows, nor did they need to range far and wide to find food and water and then travel back to family/tribe with the food and water.

Uncommon foods became commonplace, for example sugar, which used to be a rich man's pleasure due to its high cost. Meat became more tender and fatty because animals were housed to prevent movement and fed excessive food to fatten them up so that when they were sold their weight would be much higher and more profitable. There was also a shift from fish to meat, and for a long time fish was considered a poor man's food, an interesting contrast to today when global overfishing has made fish more expensive than most meat. In fact fish have even become food for farmed fish as well as supplemental protein for animals that usually don't eat fish, such as cows and sheep and chickens.

And there are also snack foods, something that didn't exist as recently as my childhood! Candies and sweets were available in my childhood, but it was still not acceptable to eat them all the time. They were strictly special treats to be eaten occasionally. Now, "snacking" is acceptable while watching TV or other sedentary activities, or for the "hunger" in between regular meals. And look at what has happened to "regular" meals. Where's Mom to cook a nutritious meal? She's probably working and does not get a chance to cook much anymore, so prepared foods can be brought into the house, e.g., pizza or McDonald's or a local eatery can be visited.

What about sweet drinks, including "fruit drinks?"

Sodas have been around for many generations and were actually used for treatment of indigestion, and soda fountains could be found at the apothecary shop or drugstore. The carbonated beverage would promote a "burp" that would make the drinker feel better and less bloated. But very sweetened soft drinks were different, and popular for their taste. As a child I would love to have Coca-Cola if I could afford it. Six ounces of very sweet carbonated water for a dime. That dime had the same purchasing power as $1 or $2 today, with which you can now buy one or two liters of sugary sodas.

I was astounded when I learned that each ounce of these sodas has almost one teaspoon of sugar! Wouldn't it still be sweet if it had half that amount?

And this is how it happens, innocently, slowly.

Continuous overeating of inexpensive tasty foods and drinks that never existed before, plus lack of physical movement, and a person changes slowly, and since everyone else is changing, too, including people in TV ads, it doesn't seem so bad to gain a "few" pounds.

I once had a pediatric patient brought to my office by his parents. He was a good-looking, well-dressed smiling little boy who appeared to be seven years old but his parents said he was five and that his problem was snoring and having sleeping problems with choking. This boy had a protruding soft abdomen and was obese. After my examination, which showed no upper airway obstruction and no enlarged tonsils, I explained to the parents that he was overweight and that was probably the main factor in his symptoms. The parents did not react too much to this and that was when I realized that both parents were quite obese, too.

How do I get obese parents to change the diet of their happy young obese boy so that he would lose weight unless they also followed a healthy program of weight loss, too? I weighed the boy and recommended a humidifier in his room and no snacks and more exercise and gave them a one-month appointment to return to my office. When they returned, I weighed the boy again and he had gained nearly two pounds. When I told this to the parents and then asked if they were feeding him less food, they told me that he was hungry all the time and they would give him bread to eat whenever he needed it. I explained that if he is hungry in between meals he should eat fresh fruit and raw vegetables like carrots.

They also said he was sleeping better with the humidifier but he was still snoring.

That clinched it for me. This was not just the boy's problem, it was the family's problem, and since this obesity epidemic was all over, it was really a national or even a global problem. Then the question for me was how to tackle this epidemic problem? The Internet is flooded with ads that tell you how to eat a healthy diet, lose weight and be happy and healthy forever, but they are all different programs, and of course many involve purchasing the "magic formula."

Anyone can look up the "blue zones" on our planet, where people can live to one hundred in good health, and try to follow their diet, and their exercise regime and lifestyle. Once you do this research, you realize that the diet can be very different from one blue zone to another, and their physical movements and exercise can vary, too. But one important factor is consistent, and that is the "real" food that these people eat, as opposed to the refined and altered food available to us and other people in areas where the obesity and diabetes epidemics are prevalent.

The climates are also different in these blue zones and the types of "exercise" performed by these healthy people are also very different from what we call "exercise" in the developed areas that make our refined foods. And then there's the stress factor, which is very high in the developed areas and low in the blue zones. Do we have to move to Greece or Sardinia or Okinawa or Costa Rica to enjoy their lifestyle, health and longevity? Obviously that would be very difficult for most people, and ultimately the influx of large amounts of immigrants to these areas would certainly change the whole picture.

What we could do is emulate the lifestyles, the diet and the physical activities of these blessed people, and maybe someday be able to get their genetics, which must also play a role in the blue zone phenomenon. Our Western lifestyle with all its stresses could be a bigger problem to solve than the diet and physical activity part. Remember that napping in the afternoon is often a part of this healthy lifestyle but would not go well with the bosses and supervisors in our fast-paced societies. The diet part is easy: more plant-based food, fresh and unrefined and non genetically modified. Avoidance of strong alcoholic beverages and sweets.

Exercise is also easy and does not have to include gyms and personal trainers.

The basic human "exercise" is walking, an activity that has been a key to our evolution and has caused us to be long-legged, upright "animals."

And the last of the three important lifestyle factors is "rest," including sleep time, napping and any other period of time when we are not working. So why is this impossible for most people living in the developed world? It would mean a complete re-orientation of our lives and society, and that would be near impossible, but we could do as much of this program as possible and enjoy the great health benefits.

It would also be helpful if the FDA, the Food and Drug Administration, would do what it is supposed to do regarding harmful or dangerous food and drug products. Historically they picture their job to involve products that would be immediately harmful, such as E. coli in meat or vegetable products, or dangerous chemicals, or plastic and metal fragments in food, but I think it's time to expand this to mean products that are harmful if used over long periods of time. There has been some progress in this area with tobacco use and alcohol. It would be nice to see that applied to processed and sugary foods and drinks.

In addition, we know that alcohol and tobacco are heavily taxed as a means to reduce excess consumption (and supply needed tax revenue for the governments who collect it), and this paradigm could be applied to the aforementioned sugary drinks. A recent attempt to do this on the local level by New York City Mayor Bloomberg was soundly defeated on the basis of jobs and traditional American freedom of choice. Well, let's think of all the other things that are taxed for our benefit along with tobacco, alcohol and now marijuana. Plus the constraints on our American freedoms that are legal, like wearing safety belts while driving in a car, which used to be voluntary and is now mandatory, or helmets for children on bicycles, which I never needed to do on my bike as a child.

We also accept speed limits while driving a car, or at least try to so we don't get an expensive speeding ticket, plus points, and we get mandatory car inspections for safety and emissions. And this list could go on and on....

The bottom line, as they say, is that it is we who are in control of our health, and not the health care system.

Chapter Eighteen - Hippocrates' Four Humors

Health is the proper balance in a living organism, be it plant or animal.

For humans we can also say that it is the condition where everything is working well, so that we are actually unaware of our physical and mental being and just enjoying life and the things we need to do and want to do. We are unconscious of the trillions of cells in our bodies that are each trying to be as healthy as possible. This near-perfect state can be considered homeostasis. Each organ, which is made up of millions and billions of cells, is in balance, constantly adjusting to all conditions so that each instantaneous stress is easily handled without our awareness.

How can this be possible?

Unfortunately I cannot answer that question, which is still part of the great mystery of life itself. Humans have been asking that question forever and there have always been healers or doctors to help them, as well as religion when there is a health stress or disease that is not readily resolved. Thousands of years ago the brilliant Greek doctor Hippocrates, the son of a doctor, surmised that each human was endowed with a strong internal "force" that could regulate health and life if there was the correct balance of four major bodily fluids, the famous four humors of antiquity: blood, yellow bile, phlegm and black bile.

At a time when there was very little medical science, this great doctor constructed an idea of how the body stayed healthy. People were smart enough to know that food and movement and rest were good natural things, so Hippocrates went one step further with the bodily humors. If there was illness that did not quickly disappear then a doctor could try to balance the humors to restore health. Blood was obviously the most important humor and the easiest to access with a knife or a leach.

A person with the right level of blood was considered sanguine, happy and comfortable. A person with a predominance of phlegm was considered phlegmatic, at peace, self-sufficient. A person with a high level of yellow bile would be considered a quick thinker, prideful, quick to action. A person with black bile predominance would be considered melancholic, introverted, thoughtful.

Remember that every person had all of these humors and was healthy when the balance was good. A doctor in ancient times could get a good idea of what illness he was treating by noting the personality of his patients. I find this paradigm is similar to modern medicine's "hormones," where health means the correct balance of all the hormones. And doctors can still get an idea of how to treat a patient by observing the personality.

The overweight man with a florid red face and trouble breathing obviously has too much blood and could be relieved by removing excess blood from his body. The results of the bloodletting would be readily noted by the patient and the doctor, and would reinforce the value of the treatment and Hippocrates' concept.

In many cases of obesity with congestive heart failure that we would now treat with diuretics, similar improvements could be accomplished with this ancient technique.

Obviously we don't have medical records from these long-ago doctors, but we can imagine that problems related to excessive yellow or black bile could be treated with emetics to induce vomiting, and purgatives (strong laxative) to rebalance the body and restore health, and likewise with treatment for excessive phlegm with peppers and snuff to induce sneezing.

Most people today have had experience with excessive phlegm at some time, with coughing and sneezing and blowing our noses to clear mucus, and many people may have noticed yellow bile while vomiting or helping someone who was vomiting, but few have seen black bile, which was probably old blood or very dark urine from hepatitis and could indicate a very serious health problem and was also associated with "dark" moods, melancholy and depression and thought to arise from the spleen.

Finally we must keep in mind the doctors' and any healers' two greatest gifts for professional success. Number 1: Most acute illness is resolved naturally. And Number 2: There is a strong placebo effect with any treatment, be it a bloodletting, an antibiotic prescription or a shaman's hand waving near your face.

Through many generations and even up to modern times, bloodletting for almost any illness was used, with mixed efficacy, but always with the placebo effect and the feeling that this was a treatment, which brings to mind the old saying, "Don't just stand there, do something!"

The ancient Egyptians may have promoted "bloodletting" when they considered menstruation as a way to expel bad blood for health reasons.

In 1799 our great president, the father of our country, George Washington was near death with a grave throat infection, suffering with fever, throat pain and difficulty breathing. He was treated by the best doctors available, and bloodletting was a major part of the treatment. It was said that the president was a great believer in bloodletting and he encouraged the doctors to do more and more of it until death finally occurred.

Today we think he may have had a Peritonsillar abscess with swelling of the throat enough to compromise his airway, and this, combined with the blood loss, killed the great man.

Finally we must admire the Oath of Hippocrates, which solidified the concept of the modern doctor who would do no harm. The doctor who would be dedicated to his patients. The doctor who would forever be grateful to the doctors who taught him how to be a doctor and consider them family, and the doctor who would keep the information about his patients' health private.

Chapter Nineteen - Health Versus Health Care

Health or health care, which would you choose?

If offered health or health care, which would you prefer? What would you answer? Health seems like the logical choice, but what if somehow you got a strange disease or had an accident, how could you manage without health insurance? Would you have left yourself open to a "no diagnosis, no treatment" scenario?

A better answer would be health with health care insurance as a backup for unpredictable events. Health actually prevents most illnesses and accidents and will make it easier to withstand unexpected illness or injury. Health and a healthy lifestyle give you the confidence to continue on the healthy path without continued reliance and dependence on a giant health care system with its frequent checkups, testing and constant changes in "health" recommendations. Interest in health is not something new, even the Old Testament's Book of Genesis gives instruction on proper diet, fruits, nuts and seeds.

There is one unspoken hazard to health insurance coverage. If you have this coverage you may be careless about your lifestyle since your insurance would cover the costs of any disease you may develop by not paying attention to healthy living.

I have been in the medical establishment for more than fifty years and have witnessed the obsession with staying "healthy," which apparently can only happen with the help of a huge health care system, as if our bodies were mere helpless slabs of meat in the face of all the illness and disease around us.

We are constantly told that the increasing life spans of the past fifty to one hundred years are proof of the wisdom of health care and its ability to prolong life. We may also be aware that the last years of many lives are spent in a twilight zone between hospital care and nursing homes.

Our society still has difficulty recognizing that "no one gets out alive" and that we should appreciate and be happy with a long and healthy life before the inevitable end, the same as all living things. Even the giant sequoia, after proudly standing for thousands of years, will fall and become food and habitat for other lives.

Thousands of years ago Hippocrates was very interested in health and recommended many things to improve health, which he thought of as an internal force in our bodies that we could nurture and strengthen through proper living, diet, exercise and rest.

We are indeed lucky to have an advanced health care system, but sadly we have neglected health. The early years of my medical career were spent treating all the problems related to smoking cigarettes, an obviously avoidable health risk. From the years of heavy smoking in America and elsewhere, a wave of cancer was met by a giant cancer treatment infrastructure and massive growth in our health care system with health insurance from employers and government.

It would be unconscionable to say we should not take care of the people who developed cancer from smoking, be it throat, lung, kidneys or all of the organs that have higher cancer rates from smoking. But why not tackle the cause and prevent the misery of cancer for the future?

Is there a similarity to the smoking plague with the plague of type 2 diabetes, with its myriad system diseases, from vision, to heart, kidneys, circulation, etcetera? Years ago in a book on diet and health by John Robbins, he compared our health care system to a hillside lookout at a beautiful countryside without a guardrail. People were continually falling over this cliff as they moved closer to the edge to get more of a view, and a squad of ambulances were ready at the bottom of the cliff to quickly transport injured and dying individuals to nearby hospitals where they received the finest supportive and reconstructive treatments, to be followed by intensive rehabilitation.

How can it be that no one thought of building a guardrail at these sites to protect the people and prevent the need for all that expensive and painful treatment. Ironically, we are sadly seeing people falling over cliffs in real time lately in overlook areas like the Grand Canyon as people strive to get the perfect selfie on their smartphone.

Today we need a guardrail to prevent the preventable diseases.

Hippocrates, Galen, Avicenna, Maimonides and other doctors of antiquity knew what the guardrail should look like. They were familiar with type 2 diabetes. The large amounts of sweet urine. No need to get into the testing method used thousands of years ago to reach this conclusion, suffice it to say that the doctors always had the "equipment" with them. Hint, it's in their mouths, but I bet they had their apprentices perform that test.

These doctors treated "well to do" clients, including merchants, clergy, royalty. Their patients had in common the ability to buy as much food as they wanted and avoid actual physical work (exercise). They gained weight, developed backaches, joint pains, chest pains, heartburn and sleep disorders along with many other chronic conditions. Their doctors would take over the kitchen, direct the diet and prescribe exercise for their patients, which might even include horseback riding. They were often rewarded with enormous fees and gifts for getting good results but may also have been punished for bad outcomes.

Poor people could not afford doctors and saw local healers, who would use herbs and possible rituals and prayer to heal. Poor people were seldom overweight, more likely undernourished, freezing in winter, conscripted to fight wars and overtaxed. Currently our American health care system costs four trillion dollars a year and rising.

A fraction of that money would be enough to really teach health and would leave lots left over to insure people against unexpected medical needs. We could also have a health care plan to reduce health insurance premiums for people who don't smoke cigarettes and people who are normal weight, and people who follow sensible exercise routines.

Remember, this would not be a program to penalize people but rather to reward people who follow healthful lifestyles which reduces health care costs and may be an incentive for people to improve their lifestyle, since monetary rewards have great power.

Years ago while in a group medical practice, several secretaries were heavy smokers who would take frequent smoking breaks throughout the day. I recommended to the doctors who I worked with that we offer a monetary prize for any of the secretaries who could stop smoking for one year. This was to be on an honor basis, but basically we could easily monitor which of the employees took smoking breaks since it was a small office and we were all friendly.

Studies have suggested that if a smoker can stop smoking for one year they will have a good chance of never smoking again. At the end of that year, one of the women won the $500 cash prize paid for by the doctors in the office. She cried and told us that the money was just the right incentive she needed to stop smoking and thanked all of us for our generosity.

Life expectancy

Our health care system is credited with increased life spans compared to the last fifty to one hundred years. My dad told me when I was a youngster that people are living longer due to advances in medical care, and that when he was growing up, people used to die in their fifties and sixties and now they live into their seventies.

I was continuously reminded of advances in medicine promoted in the news, and excited to think that I was going into such a scientific field that was curing people and prolonging life.

The first time I heard the term "three score and 10 years" applied to longevity I was at my grandmother's funeral when the rabbi giving the eulogy said she exceeded her biblical life span of three score and ten years. Apparently living to seventy may not have been the new triumph of medical science that I thought. In history class I learned that President James Madison lived to eighty-five, Thomas Jefferson to eighty-two, and President John Adams to ninety! Many of the founders of the United States also lived well past the biblical age, even considering that a four-score life span was also mentioned for stronger people. Then how did we increase our life spans so dramatically in the past fifty to one hundred years?

History shows that the deaths from World Wars I and II killed large numbers of people and this plus the virulent Spanish flu, plus the Great Depression of the 1930s dropped the life expectancy statistics dramatically. When life situations improved for most people, we were just returning to the norm of three score and ten, or four score for the strong. That still didn't explain the much longer lives of the early presidents or other historical figures around the world.

In medical school we learned about Hippocrates, the ancient Greek doctor, the father of Western medicine who gave us far more than the Hippocratic Oath, which outlined the responsibilities of the doctor. His teachings on health were as good then as any being taught today and the well-read and educated people who became our early presidents must have learned and followed his practice. He was even credited with the saying "Let food be your medicine." His teachings were carried on by the great Roman doctor Galen, a doctor for gladiators as well as Emperor Marcus Aurelius.

This medical knowledge, based on Hippocrates, was taught in colleges well into the 1800s and included diet, exercise and rest as well as bloodletting for certain ailments. Recent data on longevity in the USA shows seventy-eight years for men and eighty-one for women, which only proves that women are stronger than men, something I've always known.

A simple rule of thumb to estimate your longevity is to consider the life spans of your parents and grandparents since you share their genetics, but remember that healthy living is at least as important as genetics since we now know that "gene expression" can be positively influenced by a healthy lifestyle. Unfortunately these longevity numbers may soon drop due to the COVID-19 pandemic causing numerous additional premature deaths.

Chapter Twenty - Opioid Epidemic

Opioids are any product associated with the opium poppy or any artificial substances that are related to the opium poppy chemicals. The opium poppy has been known to mankind for thousands of years. It must've been shocking to the first people who discovered this beautiful flower with its magical properties. In the modern era, people have used these products for pain relief and for the mental effects that one gets from taking these chemicals.

Many people have seen pictures or movies that contain an opium den, where a person would rest on beds or cots and "dream" with the help of opium. Some people would continue to use opium in excess of what others used.

Can we call those people opioid addicts?

It's quite different when the addiction is to concentrated opium products such as morphine, heroin or synthetic products like fentanyl.

The ability to stifle pain was a great blessing in wartime, and opioids were used liberally during the First World War, but the practice also left us with a generation of morphine addicts. The relief of acute pain can wear off quickly and the soldier could want another dose. However the same dose may not bring the same relief as the first dose and this is common with opium products, whether it's opium itself, morphine or the numerous other opioid compounds that have been manufactured over the years.

Doctors usually paid great attention to carefully dispensing these opium products.

The dreamy and relaxed state that these products cause are also a reason why they have been used by people who did not have any pain, using it to get high!

These recreational addicts commonly paid large amounts of money to obtain the products, and this also created a criminal system where people would get the products and then sell them retail in towns or cities with a population that wanted them. There have been many restrictions on the use and availability of opium products, and people have been jailed for nonprescribed use of these chemicals. Yet people always find a way to evade these controls.

In the early part of the 20th century, you were still able to get opium-containing products without a prescription. They were treated like our present-day over-the-counter nonprescription medicines, such as aspirin or ibuprofen, but shortly thereafter availability was only from doctors treating people for pain and only by prescription.

We are born with pain-controlling mechanisms in our bodies that are activated when we are injured and feel pain. These hormone-like chemicals called "endorphins" and "endocannabinoids" will be secreted to give relief and protection to an injured or wounded person. During wartime, someone could be shot and yet not be disabled by pain and be able to escape and prevent capture or death. Even common vertebrate animals, like dogs, cats and horses have this protective system.

Pain comes in two forms. One is acute pain, for example you slip and fall to the ground and hurt your knee, and that pain may persist for hours or days, with children it may only persist for seconds or minutes. The second type of pain is chronic pain, and this can come, for example, from a displaced bone in your foot, or it could be from a strained muscle especially in the neck or lower back, and someone with this chronic pain would probably use over-the-counter painkillers such as ibuprofen, aspirin or Tylenol. They could also use physical products such as a heating pad or ice packs, which would satisfy most people with acute or chronic pain as long as the intensity of the chronic pain was manageable and not too persistent.

Someone with chronic pain would certainly enjoy a powerful painkiller such as an opioid, and the history of opioid overuse is well known to governments and to doctors.

In the United States we have an organization called the Drug Enforcement Administration (DEA) and their main function is to protect people from getting powerful drugs that they do not need and that could be dangerous to them, such as opioids.

The DEA, as it is usually called, will occasionally arrest a doctor or a group of doctors who have prescribed enormous amounts of opioids by writing prescriptions for exorbitant fees. Sometimes these people are found only after writing as many as 100,000 prescriptions, which is certainly a larger amount than would be normal to prescribe. During the recent opioid epidemic, people in some states were getting prescriptions for opioids they did not need medically and would sell them to addicts to make money to support themselves. In poor areas this was referred to as "hillbilly heroin."

When I was working with a group of internists, it was common for representatives from major pharmaceutical companies to ask to visit our offices at lunchtime to promote new medications, and they volunteered to bring lunch for the doctors. The representatives were usually friendly young women, but sometimes there would be a friendly young man. Typical drugs promoted were advanced heartburn medicines called "acid blockers" which would actually "turn off" the stomach's acid production. This was a huge advance in the treatment of "GERD" or gastroesophageal reflux disorder, mentioned in Chapter Seventeen. With this medication, people with chronic heartburn would not have to change their eating habits and could be free of discomfort, and it became a very popular new class of medications. Interestingly, the "rep" promoting this medication brought spicy pizza and soda for lunch.

We also saw "reps" who promoted blood thinners, sleep aids, erectile dysfunction meds, asthma inhalers, new antibiotics, and so on. And then one lunchtime, a young man brought hamburgers, French fries and soda and told us about a breakthrough in pain control with a slow-release opioid that was designed to prevent dependence or addiction. This was unexpected since the history of opioids was well known, at least to me as the oldest doctor in the room, but the other doctors were excited to think this was a breakthrough, just like all the other wonder drugs we were hearing about and prescribing.

I was polite and did not interrupt the speaker, but I did talk to him afterward and expressed my doubts about a nonaddictive opioid. He basically repeated his talk and emphasized the testing that was done. I spoke with the other doctors later and told them that heroin was introduced as a cure for morphine addiction and then Demerol was supposed to be a nonaddictive opioid, and that didn't work as it also turned out to be addictive. But the feedback from the younger doctors was that they had lots of patients in chronic pain who could be helped and they would try it.

It wasn't only medical doctors interested in this new opioid. Dentists involved in extractions and implants recommended this to their patients for the acute pain following their procedures. One dentist who extracted a bad molar I had, told me to take a dose of OxyContin before the local anesthetic wears off, and then another a few hours later in the day, so I would never feel any dental pain from his surgery. This did not seem like a good treatment plan and it ignored the body's own natural response to pain, plus would probably cause constipation, a well-known complication of opioids, and possibly create an addict.

These new opioids, manufactured by a well-known pharmaceutical company, became widely used throughout the United States. And although they may have helped many people with chronic pain, they created an epidemic that led to many deaths as the recreational use of this product became greater than regular medical use and "hooked" many young people, so many in fact that their unplanned premature overdose deaths impacted the life expectancy statistics of our country, just as wars had done in the past.

This epidemic is still in progress, but the manufacturers and promoters of these drugs are paying large sums of money as multiple lawsuits are being processed, and the wealthy pharmaceutical philanthropists who watched museums and hospitals place their names on their walls after they accepted philanthropic donations are now watching, with embarrassment, as these names are taken down.

This epidemic is so bad that the antidote for these opioid overdoses is dispensed for free and all first responders have it with them. Once again I have to blame the Food and Drug Administration (FDA) for not noticing this epidemic early enough, and especially the DEA (Drug Enforcement Administration), whose function is even more specific for these types of legal, powerful and life-threatening drugs. With mandatory electronic prescriptions, it should have been easier to monitor the big prescribers, as well as monitor the indications for these prescriptions.

Regarding the even bigger illegal trade in these drugs, we may need to involve an AI network that would recognize the characteristics associated with this illegal trade that continuously brings these drugs into our country by land, sea and air, even implanting these drugs inside the bodies of paid "mules" to avoid detection. And of course we must teach our children, at home and in school, the power and danger of these narcotics, and be vigilant for signs of their use.

My unexpected experience with intravenous morphine.

In my second year of medical school, I noticed right hand pain on shaking hands and felt a small, tender swelling at the base of my right palm. I didn't know the cause of this, but after a few weeks it didn't go away and I decided to go to the student health office, where a doctor could examine my hand and give recommendations for treatment. The general doctor felt my palm and noticed that I grimaced when he pressed on that spot. He wasn't sure of a diagnosis and recommended a consultation with a dermatologist.

The dermatologist I saw was also interested in how much pain I had when he pressed on this area or shook my hand, even though there was no inflammation that would indicate a possible infection. He consulted with a colleague and they came to the conclusion that I had an interesting uncommon benign tumor called a "glomus tumor," which was a vascular tumor that needed to be removed surgically. I trusted these doctors and certainly was eager to get rid of this painful growth, and I was a little excited about having an operation.

The dermatologists wanted to present my case to a class of dermatology interns and residents, so I found myself at the front of a class where the senior dermatologist would squeeze that area of my right palm so the students could see the grimace of pain that it produced and he would also demonstrate the pain of shaking hands with me. I was sent back to student health with the recommendation to get the surgery and a date was set for the operation.

The surgeon explained that I would be awake for the operation and get a different type of anesthesia called "intravenous local." For this procedure my right arm would be drained of blood for a few minutes and then a tight tourniquet would be applied to the upper arm, so that no more blood would enter the arm, and local anesthesia would be injected into the arm. The operation could be performed in about a half-hour without constant suctioning of blood from cutting into a vascular tumor.

I would be awake during surgery, and there would be very little postoperative recovery time.

On the day of the operation I waited on a bench to be called in, and though I was a little nervous, I was also hungry because I didn't have any food since midnight. I was told to lie down on the operating table and raise my right arm high. When all the blood had drained, a local anesthetic was injected intravenously into the arm and a tourniquet was applied so that no more blood could enter the arm or hand. And sure enough the operation started and I felt no pain as I laid quietly on the operating table.

After about twenty minutes I did have some discomfort in the area of the tourniquet.

The anesthesiologist must have noticed I was moving and he asked if I was having any pain and I said a little bit. I tried to continue lying still on the table and then I had the frightening feeling that I was falling off the table and shouted "stop the operation," I'm falling off the table.

The surgeon told me I was not falling and then asked the anesthesiologist what was the problem and he gave a little laugh and said, "I gave him a small dose of morphine intravenous for the pain from the tourniquet," and then the surgeon gave a little laugh, too, and when I heard this I relaxed and enjoyed the feeling of painless calm in my body.

Fifteen minutes later and the surgeon said the operation was over and he was suturing the wound and applying a dressing. The anesthesiologist loosened the tourniquet so that blood could flow into my arm again. Apparently the arm is unaffected by less than one hour of total lack of fresh blood. A few more minutes and I was transferred to a gurney and sent to recovery.

Chapter Twenty-One - Teaching

Doctors are involved with teaching and learning during their entire careers. There are always new things to learn, and medical students, nurses, interns, residents, PAs and other attending doctors are involved. This is continuous. It can be one or two minutes of teaching, like the "corridor consultation" when two doctors meet as they're walking in the hospital corridor and one has a question for the other, or formal with a teaching title, like instructor, with a planned time for teaching a targeted student audience and payment for the efforts.

I have taught medical and surgical techniques to medical students, interns and residents just as I have been taught at various points in my formal education. The most difficult for me was teaching surgery, because at some point I had to hand the scalpel to someone not as well trained as I am, and if the wrong incision is made, I am the one to blame, including legal liability. In general surgery, the operative sites are usually large, but in my specialty of otolaryngology, we often deal in small spaces that may not be well illuminated. This creates tension in the teacher and is why I didn't make this a large part of my teaching career, although I knew other doctors who were more comfortable with this practice and had less anxiety about handing over the scalpel to inexperienced students.

But I did enjoy imparting my surgical and medical wisdom acquired over more than fifty years in medicine and surgery.

It was a great pleasure and honor to convey the general and special knowledge that I had, the things I had seen and how they were treated and how the treatments had changed over the years. I enjoyed the eagerness of the younger generations to hear these things and watch how I demonstrated them, although sometimes the wisdom I had acquired conflicted with the latest recommendations that they learned in classes or from other younger attending doctors, and then they may have had to use their intellectual faculties to see that some of the older wisdom may be better than the newer recommendations. A good example of this was the "rebirth" of a procedure to improve nasal breathing.

When 1 was in ENT training all the doctors emphatically told us not to operate on the nasal turbinates except for rare exceptions because it might lead to rhinitis sicca, a condition of dry nose with crusting and poor breathing related to the enlarged open space in the nose, with evaporation of moisture that could lead to nosebleeds and possible sinus infections. But the new thinking, using advanced technology to cauterize the turbinate tissue and reduce its size for better breathing, was gaining popularity and could even be done under local anesthesia in the doctor's office. And then we started seeing a condition called "empty nose syndrome," where there was lots of objective space in the nose but the removal of too much turbinate tissue led to a sensation of poor breathing.

It turns out that a small amount of resistance in nasal breathing is important for the sensation of good breathing. It may even be needed to give the lungs resistance while breathing and may negatively affect the sense of smell, since we need a little air turbulence in the nose as the turbinates cause the inspired air to drift around, which allows scents to reach the correct intranasal spaces for optimal olfactory function. In addition, the turbinates are special paired structures with erectile tissue in the nose that can get larger or smaller to adjust the temperature and the moisture of the inspired air, a type of "high-tech" automated, climate control system.

There may be very extreme cases where giant turbinates obstruct all nasal functions, and these will obviously need surgical management. This is an example of unexpected consequences where logic may not be the answer because we don't have all the knowledge about how things work. I always cautioned the "students" about not performing unnecessary elective operations.

Doctors in training, interns and residents are very eager to operate since that seems to be the way to gain surgical proficiency, and a certain amount of operations are required to show this learning progress to the various organizations that monitor doctors' training. I reminded the students that at one time the human appendix in the abdomen was considered a useless evolutionary artifact and a source of infection that could lead to death, especially in the pre-antibiotic era. This being the case, during my surgical residency, any abdominal operation, for example removal of an infected gallbladder or a hysterectomy, could also include an appendectomy, even if the appendix was not inflamed.

The reason for this was that in the future, any abdominal distress this patient might have would not need to include appendicitis in the differential diagnosis, so the removal of this "worthless" tissue was reasonable, especially in the era when there were no CT scans or MRIs to give an exact diagnosis.

Of course today we are so much smarter and know that the appendix is an important lymphatic organ that helps to maintain the health of the digestive system and thus the whole organism. And that brings the thought that there may be other organs that we are too casual about because we don't think they are very important, and if they are "acting up" we can simply remove them.

I have always felt that all animals, including humans, have been honed into complete organisms through many years of evolution and that every part of the animal is there for a reason and removal should be very carefully considered.

In this category, for example, I include tonsils, adenoids and uterus. Recent science has suggested that the tonsils and adenoids are valuable lymphatic organs, and that removal of these organs may impair the ability to resist sinus infections, and removal of the uterus may cause structural imbalances in other abdominal organs.

Of course there are many reasons, in medical parlance, "indications," for removal of a "nonessential" organ. I have lived through a sequence of three different indications for removal of tonsils and adenoids, the first being to reduce the possibility of rheumatic fever due to persistent tonsil infections, that could ultimately lead to cardiac valve disease, and that was the era that I had my tonsils and adenoids removed at five years of age.

The next indication for removal of tonsils and adenoids in mostly children was recurrent ear infections and fluid buildup in the middle ear with conductive hearing loss, and that was a common indication during most of my private practice. The third, which is prevalent today, is to improve breathing in obstructive sleep apnea in children. I wonder if a fourth indication is lurking somewhere in the future.

A very big difference from the time I was a medical student, an intern and a resident is that today there are many more women in the medical system. At the time I was a medical student my school boasted the largest percentage of women in any medical school in the nation at about 10 percent. I also noted in my later years of practice and teaching that the women doctors and physician assistants PAs and nurse practitioners were, in general, more caring of the patients than most of their male counterparts, and often harder working, too. Unfortunately I never had the opportunity to observe the female surgeons at work in the operating room for another comparison, but I'm sure that they excel in that discipline as well.

There were some things that all the hands-on health workers that I taught, male or female, had in common. One was a large student debt burden, often six figures with high interest, and this at a time of abnormally low interest rates. Another was the lack of any "free" time during the day, since the work schedule was relentless, especially the medical record keeping, which used to be a few written lines on a paper chart and then turned into numerous lines of electronic medical record entries, most of which were not even relevant to the cases at hand.

Written records used to contain the diagnosis and the treatment, with any very interesting or unusual additional information, and this was not too time consuming. I knew many private practice doctors from my era who kept medical records on index cards.

Most of the time in a doctor-patient encounter used to be focused on the history and then the physical examination, and then the treatment options and all of this was with the doctor looking at the patient and having a back and forth dialogue. Compare that with today where the doctor or PA or NP has a computer screen in front of him or her to record all the extraneous data demanded by the medical administrators and insurance companies.

How easy is it for a patient to explain personal things to someone not even looking at them? In my private practice before EMR or electronic medical records, I would often notice things as the patient sat in front of me that were valuable in the ultimate diagnosis and treatment plan.

There are many studies that show the extra typing of electronic medical records by the "docs" is leading to work dissatisfaction and "burnout" and ultimately leaving traditional medical practice.

On a day-to-day basis I would see these hardworking health professionals "grab" a hurried lunch from the cafeteria and eat it quickly while at their workstation and then be tethered to their seats as they plowed through all the daily assigned work hoping that their computers would not fail, that they would not have to call IT to fix their computer, which would make them fall further behind in the electronic documentation. I often compared this to the administrative offices where laughter could be heard frequently, or the dining room for the administrators with freshly prepared food eaten without haste during their full lunch hour, including dessert, brought to them by hospital workers.

Who said there's no such thing as a free lunch!

Just as automation has changed most industrial work and displaced millions of workers, there are very big changes in the medical profession that were unanticipated and yet in many ways the end products of accurate diagnosis and effective treatment, which have been greatly improved.

We often don't need the highly trained and experienced physician who has seen "everything" to make a diagnosis and treatment plan, because now some young, conscientious health worker can get a decent history from a new patient, do a quick physical exam, and then order a CT scan or an MRI and lab tests, quickly get an accurate diagnosis and refer the patient to the appropriate medical or surgical specialist for treatment.

The hardest part of medicine, the diagnosis, has been made much easier.

Ultimately I foresee information technology encroachment on medical care, since "information" is what gets gathered and processed and we are already very adept at this paradigm via the giant tech companies and utilization of AI or artificial intelligence. Treatment is another issue, and it seems there will still be a need for specialist surgeons who only do one or two types of operations and become super-expert with very low complications rates. And if we ever have the courage to truly enable positive health changes in our society through the old wisdom of proper diet, exercise and rest, I fear that most doctors will need new careers.

Chapter Twenty-Two - The COVID-19 Pandemic of 2020

This is not the first, nor will it be the last pandemic that humans experience. Often called "plagues," pandemics are well documented in ancient Greece and Roman times. They are also one of the Four Horsemen of the Apocalypse.

The perfect setup for a pandemic is a large human population in a crowded environment. Other factors are extreme old age, cold weather, which puts a strain on the population, and poor health. In addition, poor diets can either create an undernourished and underweight population or an overweight and obese population, both of which are at greater risk of dying in a pandemic.

What we call "comorbidities" are another factor that promotes plagues and pandemics. A typical comorbidity could be diabetes or prediabetes, respiratory dysfunction from smoking, asthma or COPD, congestive heart failure or physical infirmities from trauma or lifestyle, which can prevent adequate exercise with reduction of fitness and immune health. Other comorbidities could be cancer or mental depression.

In ancient times, as with today, when a plague occurred those who could would leave the crowded infested areas and seek an uncrowded bucolic environment with clean air, good food and fresh water. People would naturally avoid contact with anyone who appeared ill or infirm, except in the case of close family members.

Viruses are like zombies, they are not living until they enter a living animal or plant. (Yes, plants have their own problems with viruses, too.) Once viruses invade a living organism, they redirect it to become a "factory for production of more viruses," and if they are successful they produce so many clones that they can cause an epidemic.

Should you be afraid of everyone? We should be alert, practice social distancing and wear masks in appropriate settings.

Over the years, modern people developed the concept of quarantine to get sick and contagious people away from healthy people, and even in ancient times, anyone with leprosy would be shunned and forced out of the community.

We are fortunate to have technology and resources to treat people for pandemic illness without ourselves getting infected in most cases.

Unfortunately, despite the best efforts of essential workers on the ground, our present-day pandemic has for the most part been handled improperly at the highest level and this has contributed to an excessive death toll to our population and other populations around the world.

There are about 7.8 billion people on our planet, more than three times the amount since my birth, which was really not that long ago. I don't mean to say that this pandemic occurred to curb our relentless overpopulation of our small planet, but to emphasize how many more targets for bacteria or viruses now exist compared to past pandemics, and this simple fact may explain at least some of the larger numbers of deaths from this super plague.

In addition we now have globalization and we are able to quickly travel to distant lands and fraternize with local populations, enjoy their exotic foods in their restaurants and share any dangerous viruses or bacterias that we carry, without intending to create a problem...

Furthermore, mutations are as common as life itself. Most of infectious medicine is involved in keeping up with these dangerous mutations. Take the case of penicillin. At its inception, one small fraction of a thimble full of penicillin could quickly cure many of the worst cases of pneumonia. But today the bacteria and viruses that cause pneumonia have mutated enough that we need many other types of antibiotics and antivirals to cure these infections. Likewise, with any COVID-19 treatment we may expect the same. Mutations explain why there has never been a vaccine to eliminate the common cold, also a coronavirus.

While viral mutations are something to fear, encouragingly, animals — which of course include humans — and plants also mutate to have better control of serious infections, and that's why there's never been a plague or pandemic that has wiped out our species.

I have lived through several pandemics and I have been sickened by them, too, but survived when other people were killed by them. The 1957 flu called the "Asian flu" occurred when I was a teenager in high school. I got the usual high fever, body aches and fatigue, at a time when I was young and healthy and athletic, but it did seriously impact me in a different way. I was scheduled to compete in the Westinghouse Science Competition for a prize of a paid college education. I questioned whether or not I should leave my sickbed to attend the competition or not and ultimately decided to go.

At times I was sweaty with a headache, and some questions were a strain for me. I had taken aspirin, the cure-all of the '50s, I was not in tip-top shape for the several-hour written competition but still thought I might have a chance to get one of the several prizes. Alas, I did not win but was notified that I was a fourteenth runner-up, which meant that if the other thirteen for any reason could not accept their prize, I would get it. Not much of a chance of that happening....

The next pandemic was the "Hong Kong flu" of 1968, but I never noticed that one while I was a resident in surgery working at the Queen's Hospital in Honolulu during that year.

The Swine flu in 1976 put me in bed for a couple of days with high fever and malaise and prevented me from working at my medical office most of that week. In my specialty of otolaryngology I was constantly exposed to people with throat and nose problems at close range in a time when dentists and doctors did not wear masks except in the operating room, and I was vulnerable to seasonal flu illnesses.

I finally started getting flu vaccinations but found that I would still get an occasional flu infection because it was known that the vaccines were only 50 percent to 60 percent effective. One year I had an antiviral medication on hand that needed to be taken within twenty-four hours of the onset of flu to be effective, and this expensive medication shortened my flu illness significantly.

Now the question, why is this COVID-19 so different from other pandemics we have lived through as a nation? Why so many deaths with our advanced medical industry, compared to the named flu infections above? What's different this time?

Even early on there were many sick people who treated this infection like others they had with bed rest, fluids and over-the-counter cough medicines and survived. By some estimates as many as 80 percent of the COVID infections were in this category.

We were all shocked by the astonishing number of deaths in New York City nursing homes. So many deaths occurred at once that funeral parlors and morgues were overrun, and refrigerated trucks had to be employed to hold and preserve all the dead bodies until the funeral homes could handle them. Not an inspiring sight on the streets of the Big Apple.

These elderly patients with many comorbidities were having trouble breathing and were often put on respirators which helped them breathe but did not affect the progression of the viral illness they suffered from.

At this point in medical history, medical professionals as well as the average person were all alert to treatment with antibiotics, but antiviral medications were not as commonly used. And while some patients were on ventilators, other sick people sought hospital treatment but were frequently put off due to a shortage of hospital beds, which were overwhelmingly filled with old and sickly patients with multiple severe medical conditions in addition to their new viral illness. Often those calling for help were told to stay home and only come to the hospital if they had a high fever. Unfortunately, by the time they had a high fever, they were quite sick and were also in need of a ventilator. At one point a shortage of ventilators was a crisis in itself, and estimates of a need for a million ventilators were voiced by government officials.

At no point in this crisis was the old idea of triage brought up. Triage is an old concept for prioritizing medical care in a situation where many people were at risk of dying at the same time. With limited medical personnel and facilities, people in charge needed to assess which of the injured or severely ill could survive with rapid treatment and which people were unlikely to survive with any treatment, and then use the necessary resources to save the ones most likely to survive.

Interestingly, we have been calling our fight with the COVID-19 virus a "war" since the beginning without using the concept of triage, long used in the military, until nearly a year into this battle. In a military situation after a bomb blast causing serious injury to many soldiers at the same time, triage, or prioritizing those most likely to survive in a situation with limited resources, could save many lives.

Recently there's some indication that triage has come back in the virus fight. Since the hospital beds get filled so quickly, there's no room for treatment for all COVID cases along with other emergency cases, such as automobile accidents or shootings. In these instances, tough decisions need to be made when it's obvious that some victims will not survive regardless of intensive treatment.

A shortage of hospital beds in New York City and other urban areas has occurred due to the new economics of medical care, which emphasizes more profitable outpatient care to more costly inpatient care. Decades of this practice has led to dire reductions in costly medical beds.

Everyone is shocked and terrified at all the deaths. The news media count every invaluable life lost. But are we really doing all we are capable of doing before everyone gets vaccinated?

When high-profile individuals in the government and elsewhere require hospitalization following a COVID-19 diagnosis, early in the treatment they are given approved medications to combat the virus that might otherwise kill them. These expensive medicinal cocktails, however, are not generally available to the public. While this may be due to high costs or short supply, nevertheless, not everyone has equal access to treatment. Or while seemingly everything is done for those high-status individuals, the same efforts are clearly not made for the rest of us.

Beyond these medications are preventive measures, such as public service announcements (PSAs) promoting well-known practices for improving health, especially during this time when an ominous virus is hanging over our heads. These PSAs should be placed on mainstream media, via notifications sent by text or email to people's cell phones and other devices, throughout the course of the virus.

Early COVID-19 reporting stated that nearly half of all fatalities were in overweight or obese patients and those with diabetes, which is a common finding in overweight people. Unfortunately, we did not recommend an exercise and diet weight-loss program to improve health and reduce the risk of fatal COVID illness.

Over a period of many months it would be very likely that thousands of motivated people prodded by these widely publicized health recommendations could get their BMI readings greatly improved and reduce their risk of dying from a COVID-19 infection.

In December 2020, vaccines for COVID-19 are becoming available, and this may lead to control of this pandemic. Hopefully we have learned enough from this awful pandemic to be better prepared for the next one in our future or our children or grandchildren's future.